# MOVE ON FROM SUGAR ADDICTION WITH THE SUGAR DETOX CLEANSE

## STOP SUGAR CRAVINGS: THE ULTIMATE HACK FOR APPETITE CONTROL

### GABRIELLE TOWNSEND

SILK PUBLISHING

# CONTENTS

*Introduction* ................................................................ v

1. The Emotional Aspects of Sugar Addiction ........ 1
2. Sugar Detox Cleanse Step 1 ................................. 15
3. Step 2 ...................................................................... 27
4. Step 3 ...................................................................... 40
5. Step 4 - Week 1 .................................................... 61
6. Step 5 ...................................................................... 92
7. The Detox is Done. Now What? ...................... 100

*Afterword* ............................................................. 105
*References* ............................................................ 107

# INTRODUCTION

*"Success is the sum of small efforts—repeated day-in and day-out."* — Robert Collier

Sugar is everywhere in our diets. It is present in everything from lattes at breakfast to brownies for dessert, and it is often included in every meal in between. It is easy to identify sugar when it is added to sweet treats, but it often flies under the radar and enters our diets unnoticed. Sugar hides in foods we generally perceive as healthy; the saying "an apple a day keeps the doctor away" might be true if it wasn't for the high amounts of naturally occurring sugar found in most varieties of apples. People who believe they are eating healthy may actually be consuming a great deal of sugar, and because of this, they do not understand why they struggle to maintain a healthy weight or keep potential health complications at bay.

Sugar's ability to masquerade in such a variety of forms is what makes it a health hazard to us. Despite the dangers, most people consume far too much sugar in their daily diet. Studies have found that an average American diet contains "22 to 30 teaspoons" of sugar a day, which is "considerably more than the recommended maximum of 6 teaspoons" (Santos-Longhurst,

# INTRODUCTION

2018, para. 4). But why is it that we are so prone to overindulgence when it comes to sweet things? A lack of knowledge about the real dangers sugar poses to our health, combined with the addictive nature of sugar, results in unhealthy sugar consumption habits.

Eating sugar is a vicious cycle. We often crave sugar when we are bored, stressed, or just looking for a treat to liven up our day. Eating a cookie seems like a harmless enough vice to engage in, and we get the added benefit of boosting our energy levels, however temporary that boost may be. However, after the energy boost comes the inevitable crash, and a sugar crash is especially severe. In a crash we often end up looking for more snacks, which leads us back to eating more sugar. Before long, we have become entirely dependent on sugar.

Sugar may be compelling for many of us, but can it really be called an addiction? Though cakes and cookies seem more benign than alcohol or cigarettes, they are actually just as addictive, and the term "sugar addiction" is no exaggeration. Sugar causes a dopamine spike in our brains, which temporarily boosts our moods. For people who struggle with frequent low moods and related health conditions like high stress levels and depression, this minor mood lift becomes a compulsion, and sugar becomes the main way low moods are managed. In fact, "some studies have suggested sugar is as addictive as cocaine," (Murray, 2020, para. 2). Once an addiction begins, we become more resistant to our dopamine spikes, which means we must consume more sugar to achieve the same feelings. We take larger and larger "hits" of sugar until the majority of our diet contains sugar in some form—all without realizing just how dependent we have become. This leads to higher sugar consumption and a greater risk of developing dangerous health conditions.

Additionally, like many other addictions, sugar negatively impacts your health while simultaneously encouraging you to

# INTRODUCTION

consume more and more of a dangerous substance. An addiction to sugar is a serious health concern that many people struggle with throughout their lives. High sugar levels in your body make health problems such as diabetes, high blood pressure, inflammation, and heart disease more likely to occur.

Because our bodies have become so used to our high sugar diets, it is often hard to quit sugar. It is present in a wide range of food and drinks, from fruits to alcohol to baked goods, and everything in between. We tend to naturally seek out sweet things, and trying to lower our sugar consumption makes us more likely to crave the very thing we are attempting to quit. If you attempt to cut sugar out of your diet, you may even experience symptoms of withdrawal, just as you would if you tried to stop smoking. These symptoms can include more intense cravings, nausea, mood swings, and fluctuating energy levels.

Despite these difficulties, it is incredibly important to replace a diet high in sweets with one that is good for your body and your mind. Ending your sugar addiction is one of the best things you can do for yourself. Your health depends on your ability to moderate the presence of sugar in your diet.

## THE IMPORTANCE OF KICKING YOUR SUGAR HABIT

Sugar is much more dangerous than its sweet taste implies. While sugar tastes great and our bodies may crave it, the excessive sugar levels in most Americans' diets does them no favors. Sugar is one of the leading causes of obesity. If you're having trouble managing your weight, you should review just how much sugar you're really eating. It also commonly leads to inflammation and high blood pressure. Together, these conditions can drastically increase the likelihood of more serious health problems. They cause your cardiovascular system to struggle to keep up with your body's needs, which puts strain on your heart and your arteries. If left unchecked, this can

# INTRODUCTION

develop into heart disease, which can be a life-threatening condition.

Kicking a sugar habit is hard, but with the right information and the right plan, you can increase your chances of successfully lowering the amount of sugar in your diet. You do not have to be controlled by your cravings any longer. Your sugar addiction will be a thing of the past. With the help of this book and the steps outlined in the sugar detox cleanse, you can improve your meal habits, routinely make healthier choices, and begin the journey towards a healthier life.

I know firsthand the dangers of sugar, which is why I am so committed to providing you with the best possible plan for ending your sugar addiction. Food was a coping mechanism for me in my youth. I used sugary snacks as an outlet for my struggles in my personal life, and as a result, I struggled with obesity and developed type 2 diabetes at just 35 years old. I knew I had to make a change, and I needed to make one that would last, or my health would be in serious danger. By learning healthier coping mechanisms and developing better nutrition habits, I lost over 200 pounds in three years. I also developed healthy habits that have stuck with me every year since. I want to show you how to make changes in your diet, especially in regards to sugar, that will support the development of a more positive relationship with food.

It is time to stop letting sugar control you. Whether you are trying to prevent future health issues or you need to make changes to your diet to manage health conditions that have already developed, the sugar detox cleanse can help you beat your not-so-sweet addiction. This book will provide you with a better understanding of why sugar is such a difficult addiction to quit, as well as steps anyone can use to remove excessive sugar from your diet. By moving on from your sugar addiction, you can improve your relationship with food as a whole and support a healthier lifestyle.

# 1

# THE EMOTIONAL ASPECTS OF SUGAR ADDICTION

## WHY GIVING UP THE SWEETS IS SO HARD

Sugar is notoriously hard to quit. Many people who try to eat less sugar find themselves falling back into old habits, regardless of how many reasons there are to minimize its presence in our diets. This may even be something you have attempted previously before with little success. You may be tempted to chalk it up to just how many foods we eat every day that contain sugar —it is present in everything from fruit, to candy, to bread and pasta, which can make it hard to avoid. However, this doesn't fully account for the power of sugar's temptation and the frequency of sugar cravings when compared to many other types of food. After all, people quit eating certain foods all the time, even those which make up a great deal of a standard diet. People who develop gluten intolerance or celiac disease cut out bread and find replacements to make all their meals gluten-free. Becoming vegan or vegetarian means removing many meat products from your meal plans. You could probably stop eating some less popular foods like Brussels sprouts and chard without too much difficulty. What is it about sugar that makes it so difficult to cut out of your diet?

Sugar's power over us is a result of its connection to our

emotions. Unlike many foods, our consumption of sugar has a direct impact on our brain chemistry. Rather than just filling us up, sugar makes us feel happier. It releases dopamine in our brains, and when we get that dopamine rush we become compelled to seek it out more and more often. We are constantly seeking out the source of momentary happiness that sugar provides, and the longer we spend chasing our "sugar high," the more sugar we must consume to get the same result. Think of how you consumed candy as a kid. It is very likely that back then, only a piece or two of chocolate was enough to send you into a sugar rush. Your brain responded much more strongly to the presence of sugar because it was a minimal part of your diet. Now, however, the same amount of sugar isn't likely to have you bouncing off the walls; it may not have an effect on your mood at all. Instead we must eat much more sugar to get the same results, which only makes it harder to end our sugar addictions. The more sugar we eat, the more change we would need to make to our eating habits to end our dependence on sugar.

Addiction to sugar is especially strong for those struggling with mental health and mood issues, and it is especially hard to quit as a result. You might be unknowingly using sugar as a way to cope with negative emotions. Many people who have experienced traumatic events or who suffer from depression and anxiety reach for sweet snacks when they are reminded of a negative event. Sugar makes us feel happier, and it can even balance us out when we enter an emotionally volatile state. The boost from sugar makes it easier to bring your mood back up, but it also means that you are managing your mood in a dangerous way. Continued use of sugar to regulate your emotions can lead to many health problems as sugar consumption gets out of hand.

Sugar dependency is comparable to an eating disorder, and it is often a component of stress eating and binge eating. Food serves as a way to calm your nerves, improve your mood, and manage other unfavorable factors in your life. You may feel a compulsion to eat when you are having trouble handling a recent development and your emotional state suffers. However, overindulging and eating the wrong things leads to health scares, especially when what you are eating has a high sugar content. It is harder and harder to end this behavior because eating sugar makes you feel good, while restricting your cravings gives you no such immediate gratification. While you may feel better in the long run if you end these behaviors, managing them in the short-term can leave you feeling unmotivated, lacking energy, and flip-flopping between emotional extremes.

This is the harmful and potentially even deadly trap of sugar. Under the sweet veneer lies a dangerous substance that is highly addictive because it preys on emotional vulnerability. It is so easy to become addicted to sugar because it seems like a relatively harmless addiction compared to others, but in reality the many hidden dangers and the cycle of dependence it creates can keep you trying to kick your sugar habit for years if you don't have the right strategy.

## SIGNS YOU'RE ADDICTED TO SUGAR

You might eat sugar fairly regularly, but is the situation really so out of control? How do you know if you're addicted to sugar? Some people consume sugary foods as an occasional treat without feeling a strong desire to continue eating it, while others develop a real addiction. Of course, everything is fine in moderation, but the key defining trait of a sugar addiction is that moderation becomes impossible. You may be addicted to sugar if you experience any of the following behaviors and thought patterns.

*You Crave Sugary Snacks Constantly*

In one way or another, sugar is always on your mind. In

much the same way as smokers are often thinking about their next cigarette, you are near-constantly thinking about the next time you can have sugar. This may be a craving for something sweet in general, or it may be a desire for a particular sugary comfort food that you have come to associate with improving your mood. Whatever shape your personal sugar craving takes, the only time it is not occupying your thoughts is when you are currently indulging in it.

Though sugar cravings may be persistent, this doesn't mean that they are always recognizable. Some cravings may lurk under the surface, and only when you begin to feel bored or snackish do you immediately default to looking for something sweet. You can focus on other, more important things in the meantime, but that desire for sugar sits at the back of your mind and strikes at its first opportunity.

Constant cravings can lead to irregular eating habits. Ideally, you should be eating your meals around the same time each day. Snacking heavily in between, or taking meals at odd hours as a result of powerful cravings, completely throws off your daily meal schedule. You may find yourself having more late-night snacks, or waiting to eat dinner until very late because you spent the day snacking. Without regular meal times, you will find yourself feeling hungry nearly all the time, which can worsen the compulsion to overeat.

*Bad Moods Make Your Cravings Worse*

Because sugar has such a strong impact on your emotional state, you begin to associate eating sugar with feeling happier. This causes you to seek a solution for a bad mood in the form of sugar. When your mood dips and you start to feel agitated, you get a powerful desire to eat something sweet. This may be a conscious thought, or you may find yourself unconsciously snacking or reaching for a sugary drink. The compulsion to use sugar to handle a bad mood furthers your dependency on sugar, worsening the addiction. Your brain correlates feeling good with eating sugar and you start seeking it out to remedy even minor mood dips. When you are denied sugar, your mood falls even further, leading to more frequent bouts of irritability.

Though sugar provides a temporary mood and energy boost, it is not long-lasting, and it does little to deal with the reasons behind your bad mood. It's like slapping a bandage over the problem without dealing with the actual injury. You may feel a bit better in the moment, but whatever caused that bad mood will not be fixed. Negative thoughts that are a product of mental health issues or trauma will continue to persist without being adequately addressed. By quelling the thoughts with sugar, you simultaneously increase their frequency and lower the likelihood of seeking out better coping strategies for these mood swings.

*You Eat Even When You Are Not Hungry*

When you are addicted to sugar, you start seeking out sugar as often as possible. This means that you will often snack between meals. If you don't have much to do, you might head for the fridge or pantry and take a look around. Eventually, you start to eat whenever you are bored or looking for a small boost, which means you might be snacking near-constantly throughout the day.

You may be driven to eat, especially sugary foods, because you aren't able to find an outlet for certain issues. Low energy and boredom are common triggers, both of which can be solved in different ways. When you choose to eat instead of finding another, healthier method for revitalizing yourself, you encourage your own reliance on sugar.

*You Frequently Engage in Overeating*

As mentioned above, eating more often and seeking out food when you aren't hungry is a gateway to overeating. Overeating is very difficult to stop once you start. This is because you are essentially training your stomach to accept and crave more food than you would otherwise need. When you overeat, your stomach expands to make room for the food; this is why you may feel bloated, distended, and uncomfortable when you eat too much in one sitting. When binge eating occurs on a regular basis, you increase the capacity of your stomach gradually over time. This means you are hungry more often and you must eat more to satisfy your hunger. It is very hard to lose weight and manage your eating habits at this point because you can no longer have smaller meals and feel satisfied. This only leads to more overeating, starting the cycle anew.

After overeating, you may feel very sluggish as your body attempts to digest everything. This is especially true of high-carb meals, and as you may know, carbs are just more complex forms of sugars that are broken back down into simple sugar molecules in your body. It takes energy to break these molecules down, which is why you might feel so tired after a big bowl of pasta. Even though sugars provide your body with energy, that energy is often short-lived and the crash is typically worse than the initial energy boost. Additionally, many carbs contain tryptophan, which is an amino acid that can cause you to feel drowsy. Eating sugar traps you in a cycle of overeating, energy fluctuations, and often guilt as a result of your inability to control your eating habits.

*You Experience Sugar-Related Health Problems*

Sugar is a perfect example of how having "too much of a good thing" can be very harmful. While a little sugar in moderation is fine, eating too much sugar on a regular basis increases your likelihood of developing various health problems. One of the most notable health concerns related to sugar is the tendency for spikes and dips in your blood sugar. An instability in your blood sugar can make you tired more often, and it can put you in a bad mood more frequently, which just causes you to seek out sugar once again. The hormone responsible for managing your blood sugar level in your body is called insulin. When functioning normally, insulin removes and stores excess energy in the form of glucose, or sugar, from your bloodstream and moves it into your cells. However, when we eat excessive amounts of sugar, the insulin receptors in your cells start ignoring the presence of this hormone. This is a condition known as insulin resistance. It is a precursor to many more troubling health conditions that occur because your body can no longer process the sugar you eat. These health conditions include strokes, heart disease, and type two diabetes.

Type two diabetes is a particularly concerning health condition that can affect your life for years to come. It develops as a direct result of insulin resistance. Your body responds to your cells' inability to use insulin by producing even more insulin in your pancreas. The role insulin is meant to fulfill is not getting completed, so your body doesn't know how else to react other than to redouble its efforts. Eventually, your pancreas cells get worn out from the overproduction and can't keep pace, which means your insulin levels start to sharply drop. This results in a rise in your blood sugar that ultimately develops into type two diabetes when not appropriately addressed (Harrar, 2019, para. 4). By the time you are diagnosed with diabetes, insulin resistance has been occurring for a long time. It is merely the product of months or years of sugar addiction.

Another health condition that may develop as a result of too much sugar in your diet is metabolic syndrome. This is not just one health problem, but instead it represents a large group of related health issues, many of which have very few symptoms and can linger under the surface until more severe conditions develop. Metabolic syndrome includes high blood sugar, high blood pressure, high cholesterol, and excess body fat, especially around the waist area. These smaller problems build to form a much more dangerous whole. They can lead to grave health issues that threaten your ability to lead a healthy and happy life.

. . .

*A Lack of Sugar Brings Bad Moods*

When our emotions are tied to our sugar consumption, it is only natural that a lack of sugar will bring on bad moods more frequently. If you are addicted to sugar, you will become irritable if you go too long without any sugar or if you don't have enough sugar in a period of time. You may find yourself seeking it out to deal with these moods, and when you do get some sugar, you will associate the alleviation of your bad mood with the sugary snack or drink.

Because sugar is an addiction, attempting to abruptly cut it out of your diet can highlight just how dependent on it you have become. Many people have even said that trying to quit sugar led them to experience symptoms that were similar to withdrawal. You may feel more powerful cravings, more frequent mood swings, and physical malaise all because your body is not getting the amount of sugar it is used to.

## SUGAR DETOX

An addiction to sugar is more powerful than you may anticipate. You might believe that cutting sugar out of your diet is as simple as having the willpower to avoid that cupcake or slice of pie at the next party, but the truth is much more complicated than that. You have likely spent years building up a dependency upon sugar, so when you abruptly try to remove it, your body will react to the sudden loss. Like any addiction, you will start to experience moderate to severe withdrawal symptoms.

During sugar detox, your body protests against the shift in your eating habits. It is used to getting an excess of sugar, and depriving it of sugar very rapidly means that you will experience powerful cravings for its return. You are likely to also experience fluctuations in your energy levels, more common bad moods, and a higher frequency of headaches and stomachaches. Though these symptoms can be intimidating, they are well worth the benefit of no longer being tethered to sugar.

*Lack of Energy*

Sugar provides you with energy, but it also frequently results in energy crashes. To avoid this, you may have steadily increased the amount of sugar you ate over time so that there was rarely a moment where sugar wasn't providing you with energy. Because of this, you are likely unaware just how dependent you are on sugar for your usual energy levels. If you suddenly cut sugar out of your diet, you will heavily experience those energy crashes that you were minimizing through your sugar cycle.

Low energy is difficult to deal with, and it can seriously harm your motivation to stick to your sugar detox cleanse. When you are tired, you only want to give in to your cravings, and you lose the energy you would need to fight them. You think about how much easier it would be to go back to eating sugar, but you forget all of the reasons why you are committing yourself to ending your relationship with sugar in the first place. If you find yourself experiencing low energy, fuel yourself with more nourishing, healthier sources of energy instead. Choose foods that will keep your motivation high and that give you a long-lasting boost without any of the crash. Replacing sugar with these kinds of foods helps you maintain a balanced state of energy rather than the constantly fluctuating version that sugar provides.

*Poor and Fluctuating Moods*

As previously discussed, sugar makes us feel happier because it causes our brains to produce more dopamine. When we take away the sugar, we also take away these dopamine spikes. This can result in more frequent bad moods with no easy fix. You may find yourself more easily irritated and more prone to bursts of sadness and frustration. You may also find that you have little patience for minor annoyances that were tolerable before. This can cause you to lash out at others or to turn your negative thoughts inward.

A poor mood is difficult to manage in the moment, but it is only temporary. The longer you go without giving in and appeasing your mood with sugar, the more you will learn to regulate your mood through healthier methods. You may find that engaging in a relaxing activity like reading or watching some television soothes your nerves just as effectively. Alternatively, you might be someone who uses exercise as an outlet for frustrations. Giving yourself a positive outlet for these feelings is very important, not just for your relationship with sugar but also for your relationship with your mental health. Eventually, you will get dopamine spikes from these healthy alternatives instead, and you will no longer be waiting for your next taste of sugar to even out your emotions.

*Insomnia*

Sugar usually keeps us up at night, and yet, cutting sugar out of your diet can lead to temporary insomnia. This seems counterintuitive at first, but one possible explanation ties back to the energy spikes and crashes that sugar causes. When you give up sugar, you no longer experience the severe crashes that can make you very tired very suddenly. If you once relied on these crashes around bedtime, you may find that you have more difficulty falling asleep, at least for a short while after quitting.

Sooner or later, your body will begin to regulate itself to your usual sleeping patterns without the use of sugar crashes. This process is made easier by waking up at a certain time each day and getting ready for bed at a certain time each night. The longer you stick to this schedule, the more your body will find a rhythm of getting tired at a certain time, and the easier it will be to fall asleep at night to get the rest you need.

*Intense Cravings*

Cravings are very common when you quit sugar. They are one of the most powerful forces encouraging you to give up on your attempted detox. Cravings may be minor at first, but they can quickly develop into major problems if you don't find something to replace them with. When you crave sugar, swap out the snack for something sugar-free that you can feel good about eating and that you also enjoy. This is a similar idea to smokers who quit by chewing gum every time they get the craving to smoke. You can also minimize cravings by making sugar difficult to access in your house. Having sugar readily available makes it harder to resist the temptation to just open the pantry and grab something. If you need to go all the way to the store to get something sweet, you are more likely to settle for a substitute instead.

*Digestive Problems*

Sometimes the sugar detox can cause digestive issues. Any big change in your diet can throw your digestive system off, and cutting out sugar is no exception. You may experience an upset stomach or a fluctuating appetite. Either issue can complicate your relationship with food further and make it harder to settle into a sugarless diet.

To minimize digestive issues, you might consider adding more probiotic foods to your diet. Probiotics support healthy gut function and make stomach problems less frequent. Yogurt is a popular choice, but if you prefer you can choose to take probiotic supplements instead. You should also minimize the presence of any foods that worsen your upset stomach in your meals. The specific foods that bother your digestive system may vary, but foods high in saturated fats like fried foods are a common source of upset stomach. Spicy foods can cause similar issues, as can dairy. Once your stomach is feeling more stable, you can start reintroducing these foods back into your diet, but cutting them out for a short time alongside sugar can save you some trouble.

*Light-Headedness and Dizziness*

A lack of sugar, combined with the resulting lack of immediate energy, can occasionally leave you feeling light-headed and dizzy. When your energy fluctuates and dips, you can feel a bit disoriented. More often than not this is a fleeting feeling that isn't much cause for alarm. If you feel light-headed, rest and wait for the sensation to pass. Lying down can help your body shake the dizzy feeling.

While light-headedness often goes away on its own after a brief period, a prolonged period of dizziness can be cause for concern. If you have diabetes or you are at a risk of developing diabetes, dizziness can be a symptom of low blood sugar. The light-headedness occurs because your body does not have enough sugar in your bloodstream to maintain proper brain function. In these cases, you may need to consume a bit of sugar until you are feeling better, though be sure to limit your sugar intake to a healthy amount.

## A GRADUAL ADDICTION

When dealing with sugar, it is important to note that it isn't the type of addiction that occurs after just one taste. It can take years of consuming excess amounts of sugar before you are really addicted to it. Because of how gradually the addiction develops, it can sneak up on you, and learning the full extent of the damage sugar has done is quite a shock. You might not even realize there is a problem until you try to lower your sugar intake, at which point it becomes apparent just how thoroughly dependent on sugar you have become without even noticing it.

Sugar's ability to lurk silently in many things you eat each day only contributes to how difficult sugar addictions are to identify. If you don't typically check nutrition information labels, you may be unaware just how much sugar is in a certain snack or meal. Just because something doesn't taste very sweet doesn't mean there is no sugar to be found in it. Neglecting to read the ingredient list can leave you unaware of sugar's presence in a variety of foods. Sauces are an especially heinous culprit of this crime, as they tend to contain very high amounts of sugar while still being savory rather than sweet. This tricks your taste buds while still flooding your system with sugar. Another example that is particularly detrimental is salad dressing. While not every dressing has a high sugar content, many of them do. If you don't read the label, you could believe you are making yourself a healthy lunch when in reality you are just pouring sugar on top of your salad. A greater awareness of sugar hiding in plain sight can make it easier to avoid unnecessary sugars and choose healthier options.

Once you start thinking of sugar as an addiction, you will find yourself looking back on past behaviors in a whole new light. If you're an emotional eater, you may not consider the damage of what you are doing until long after it has been done. You might hardly notice you've opened a package of cookies until you are nearly finished with them, at which point guilt is often quick to follow. When you make an effort to become more aware of your sugar consumption, you become better at spotting potential emotional triggers for eating. You can then regain control over them before they can negatively impact your health.

*Taking Back Control of Your Diet*

Decreasing your sugar intake is all about having a better sense of control over what you are eating. While beating a sugar addiction isn't easy, the sense of self-discipline and fulfillment you will gain from the process is worth every headache and craving you experience in the process. The improvements in your health are immediately noticeable, and you will save yourself from many future health conditions just by altering your diet. Additionally, you will feel a sense of accomplishment in seeing just how strong your desire and willpower really is.

People who successfully complete a sugar detox feel great about themselves and their choices. They know they have made a positive change in their eating habits that will benefit them from years to come. Many people who complete this process never go back to their old eating habits because they have learned the skills to control what they eat and have discovered many healthy alternatives to sugary foods. The following chapters will provide you with the tools and knowledge you need to make this change for yourself. They will guide you through every step of the process so that you can experience your own sugar detox cleanse success story and never look back.

## 2

# SUGAR DETOX CLEANSE STEP 1
## IDENTIFY YOUR FOOD TRIGGERS

The sugar detox is not a slow, gradual reduction of the number of carbs you eat. When you ease yourself into the process, you leave yourself open to many opportunities for slip-ups. It is easier to reach for a candy bar because you've decided that some sugar is okay. It is also easy to not realize just how much sugar you are consuming if you only take small steps to get rid of it very slowly. You can find yourself eating far more than you intended because those sources of temptation are all around you. Additionally, it takes much longer to see or feel the effects of removing sugar from your life. If you go a few days and nothing seems different, you may get discouraged and inhibit your progress, getting stuck in this process for months instead of the week or two you had initially planned. Worse, you may lack the motivation to continue and find that your cravings are too strong because you are still frequently satisfying them. This can make you give up on the diet altogether.

You want to avoid giving yourself opportunities to sneak sugar into your diet. This is why the cold turkey approach of the sugar detox cleanse is the best way to start shifting your dietary habits in a way that will produce long-lasting change. The first step is to get rid of the foods you know you shouldn't be eating. If you rid your cabinets, pantry, and refrigerator of all the foods that will tempt you into ending your sugar fast, it is much harder for you to cheat on your diet, and you will increase the likelihood of success.

While it is a good idea to get rid of all sugary foods, take special care to remove your most common food triggers. If you have a weakness for soda, make sure there is none in the house when you start your detox. Don't trust that you will be able to limit yourself to just one occasionally; more often than not, when you have gone a few days without sugar, the allure of a can of soda is stronger than you anticipated. You want to stay strong during this first week of detoxing. If you show yourself that you can make it through a week without sugar, it will be easier to stick to a low sugar diet in the future. Set yourself up to succeed by throwing out the things in your cabinet that will interfere with a sugar-free lifestyle.

## FOODS TO ELIMINATE DURING DETOX

The list of foods that contain high amounts of sugars, especially added sugars, is very long. You may be surprised to see some items on the list, as their sugar content is well hidden under many other flavors. Oftentimes you do not think of these high-sugar items as "sweet," but they can interfere with your progress, nonetheless.

Work your way through all the food in your house with this list in hand. Remove anything that appears on the list, as well as anything else that contains high amounts of sugar. It may be sad to feel like you are wasting these items, but what you lose in wasted purchases you more than make up for in the benefits of living a healthier lifestyle free from the shackles of sugar. You will not regret cleaning your pantry and fridge of these foods that pose a threat to your well-being. You will be glad you did it when you start to see the results that come from cutting out sugar. Eliminating these foods from your household early on means they will not tempt you later down the line when cravings start hitting the hardest.

## Desserts

In a sugar detox, all kinds of sweet and savory desserts have to go. Anything that includes chocolate, specifically milk chocolate, already has a high amount of added sugar and should be disposed of. Chocolate can cause powerful cravings, so it is especially important that it is not around to tempt you. This means eliminating all chocolate treats and candies. You should also rid yourself of any cookies, cakes, cupcakes, and baked goods in your house. Ice cream is equally sugary, as is frosting. These desserts don't do you any favors, and their overly sweet taste worsens sugar addiction.

Don't be fooled by desserts that seem to taste less sweet but are still packed with sugar. Something like pound cake, for example, can at first seem like a healthy replacement for regular cake. It is true that with pound cake there is no sugar-filled icing to worry about, which is one of the worst offenders on a sugar detox. However, there is still plenty of sugar in the refined white flour used to bake the cake, and many pound cakes have a sweet glaze on top. If you take a look at the label, you will see just how deceptively sugary even pound cake can be. This is true for a number of seemingly innocuous desserts, so use a critical eye when evaluating desserts and when in doubt, throw it out.

*Prepackaged and Boxed Meals and Snacks*

Prepackaged meals are another big offender of high sugar content, though they are a much less obvious source of sugar than desserts. You might not think that the frozen meal you are microwaving could possibly contain that much sugar, but prepackaged meals almost always have added sugar in some form to improve the taste after sitting on a freezer shelf for months. Additionally, these kinds of meals are full of preservatives whether they are expected to stay frozen for a long time or if they are self-stable for months or even years. These preservatives don't do your health any favors either. It is better to learn how to make fresh versions of these kinds of meals where you can control exactly what goes into them.

Another shelf-stable item to worry about are the various boxed snacks available to you at the grocery store. These could be chips, crackers, cookies, or any number of items, but the one unifying trait is that nearly all of these kinds of snacks will have high sugar content. Check the nutrition label of these foods as you take them out of the pantry and note just how many grams of carbohydrates, which your body breaks down into sugar, are in a handful of *Cheez-Its*. Hidden carbs are just as dangerous as more obvious sources of sugar, if not more so. If you are not careful about your eating habits, having a few crackers could have the same sugar impact as eating a whole spoonful of icing.

Despite their marketing as healthier snacks, granola bars are also full of added sugars. Many granola bars include chocolate chips, drizzle, or a chocolate base, especially those marketed towards kids. Others have sugary additives like marshmallows, honey, maple syrup, corn syrup, dried fruit, and many more hidden sources of sugar. It's a good idea to steer clear of granola bars in general, as they tend to use added sugar to balance out the flavor of the oats. If you really want to include them as an easy to eat snack, check both the nutrition information and the ingredients list for how high they are in added sugar. Stick to whole-grain options and ditch anything that prioritizes flavor over health benefits.

*Sweetened Beverages*

Sweetened beverages are many people's kryptonite. Soda is an especially notable offender, as it is so widely available and many people started drinking it in their early adolescence—building a habit young. Soda is one of the worst things you can keep in the house if you are trying to quit sugar. You may think diet soda would be a good replacement, but it is usually better to quit soda altogether. Diet soda is still not good for you, even if it doesn't have sugar or calories. In fact, because it seems like a healthier choice, you may end up drinking more diet soda than you ever did regular soda, which doesn't do your body any favors.

Of course, soda is not the only beverage that can contain tons of sugar. You would be surprised by just how high in sugar some supposedly healthy beverages actually are. Fruit juices tend to have a great deal of sugar, both naturally and from added sweeteners. Sports drinks and vitamin water also pack a shocking amount of sugar. While it may serve as an energy boost for athletes, it isn't a healthy amount of sugar to be adding into your diet on a regular basis. Many flavored waters are sugar-free, but others are far from it, so don't be fooled by the implication that all of these drinks are safe to consume. The best thing to drink will always be water, but there are still many drinks that do not contain added sugars that you can use to replace these sweet beverages in your diet. Sparkling water is a great substitute.

*Refined Carbs*

Not all carbohydrates are created equal. While complex carbs are okay to eat on a low-sugar diet, refined carbs, also known as simple carbs, should be avoided. We will talk about complex carbs in more detail in future chapters. For now, it is enough to know that refined carbs have largely been stripped of many of the health benefits that complex carbs provide. They also are almost always packed with added sugar in the baking process, which makes them a danger to your detox.

. . .

The list of refined carbs is long and contains many different foods. In general, it includes bready products that are not made with whole grains and anything made using white flour. This includes white bread, pasta, any pastries and cakes, dough, buns, and breakfast items like cereal, pancakes, and waffles. White rice is also a refined carb, as is rice flour made from white rice. If you want to stick to your sugar detox, you should eliminate all of these sources of simple carbs from your kitchen.

Refined carbs are an especially negative influence on your diet because it is hard to recognize them as being unhealthy. When you think of sugar, pasta isn't usually the first thing to come to mind. Despite this, refined carbs can be just as harmful as more obvious sources of sugar when consumed in excess. Consider refined carbs as "processed carbs" and avoid them as you would other unhealthy processed foods. Take care not to allow these refined carbs to slip past your radar when cleaning out your pantry.

*Sweet Sauces and Dressings*

If you want to have healthier meals, limit the amount of sauces, dressings, and dips you use. The vast majority of sauces and dressings contain sugar to improve the flavor and balance out the acidity of common ingredients like tomatoes and mayonnaise. Ketchup, one of the most common condiments, is loaded with sugar. You may think that you are only using a tiny amount of these sauces so they don't pose an issue, but the sugar content can add up every quickly and stall your progress on the sugar detox.

Despite the risks they pose, not every sauce is as sugary as some of the worst offenders. Dressings that are mostly oil-based, and carb-free sauces that don't have any added sugars, can still be incorporated into your diet. For example, hot sauce and buffalo sauce are almost always low- or no-carb, and they can add a spicy kick to a plain meal. If spice isn't your thing, balsamic dressings, ranch, and yellow or brown mustard all make for great sugar-free options.

*Cereal*

If you're looking to make yourself a healthy breakfast, leave cereal out of the picture. Most cereals are made with white flour, which means they are refined carbs with little nutritional value. These only add sugar into your diet, which might make you a little more energized in the morning, but which will inevitably lead to a crash later in the day. Many cereals also add sweet ingredients like chocolate, honey, marshmallows, dried fruit, and artificial flavorings that make them especially unhealthy.

Some cereals avoid these pitfalls and manage to provide a good source of healthy carbs without all of the added sugar. These are typically multigrain cereals that are marketed more towards adults rather than the colorful, sugary options meant to attract kids' attention. While they may seem a bit "boring" compared to *Lucky Charms*, whole grain cereals with minimal added ingredients can be a good replacement if you are used to starting your days off with sweeter options. Just be sure to check the label for any unwanted sweeteners.

*Flavored Yogurt*

Yogurt is almost always held up as a healthy snack, but the truth is that many yogurts are not healthy at all. The flavored yogurts you see advertised on TV or displayed to pull your attention in the store may be more exciting than plain options, but they are also far higher in sugar. Added fruit and flavorings minimize the health benefits you could otherwise receive from yogurt and turn a nutritious snack full of probiotics into spoonfuls of sugar.

Instead of buying pre-made flavored yogurts, cut up a bit of fruit and add some healthy whole grain granola to plain yogurt yourself. This allows you to control how much sugar goes into your snacks while also ensuring that any sugar comes from natural sources rather than artificial ones.

*Canned Soup*

Canned soup frequently contains surprisingly high amounts of sugar. Sweetness is used as a way to improve the flavor of any shelf-stable product. Additionally, soups commonly use many ingredients that are high in sugar. Those with pasta noodles or rice contain refined carbs, as do soups containing dumplings. On the whole, if you are really in the mood for soup, it is better to make it yourself. Not only will you avoid all these sources of sugar, you will also have a big batch of leftovers you can use for quick and easy meals throughout the week to help your snack habits.

Canned soups are also very high in sodium, which poses health problems of its own. A high sodium diet puts you at a greater risk for having high blood pressure. When your blood pressure is high, you increase your risk for heart disease, heart attacks, and stroke. As many as "1 in 3 Americans will develop high blood pressure in their lifetime," largely as a product of the number of processed foods in the standard diet (Cox, 2013, para. 8). Dropping canned soup from your meal rotation targets two sources of health risks and improves your overall health.

*Dried Fruits*

Any snack that includes fruit is theoretically better for you than more traditionally unhealthy options like cookies, but not when you consider the sugar content. Fruits often contain far too many sugars to be consumed in large quantities. The sugars occur naturally, yes, but your body metabolizes them in the same way, and eating too much fruit can still be bad for your health. It is best to only have fruit as an occasional snack and to try to choose fruits that are lower in sugars.

Dried fruits are also worse for you than regular fruits because they often contain great quantities of additional sweeteners. Sugar is added to fruits in the drying process to improve flavor, alongside many preservatives to keep them tasting fresh while still being shelf-stable. If you're really in the mood for fruit, skip the added sweetener and just buy a carton of berries or another low-sugar fruit to satisfy your cravings.

*Jellies and Jams*

Peanut butter and jelly sandwiches may be a childhood staple, but they are not quite as good for you as you may think. Jellies and jams should be avoided for many of the same reasons as dried fruits. They contain fruits that are naturally high in sugar and can pose a risk to your health. This is despite jellies and jams typically being seen as a healthier option than other toast spreads like butter or margarine. Sugar is often added in the preserving process, which only increases the sweetness of these products. Steer clear of these and other fruit preserves to avoid the high amounts of sugar present in just a teaspoon or two of jam or jelly.

*Sugar and Sweeteners*

If you're on a sugar detox, it is obviously a good idea to avoid adding sugar to anything you make or eat. This includes adding sugar to your morning coffee, sprinkling it over fruit, or using it to sweeten up a dish. You should also avoid brown sugar, as it poses the same health risks as regular white sugar with added molasses.

Many sweeteners have gained popularity recently as healthier alternatives to sugar, but don't be fooled by these claims. While some sweeteners are indeed zero-calorie, zero-sugar healthy options, others are replacements that do nothing to lessen the negative health impacts, and in some cases are worse than just using regular sugar. High fructose corn syrup, for example, is an additive in many different foods, but it is typically considered to be less healthy than sugar. Honey is similarly full of sugars, and while it is certainly better for you than corn syrup, it should also be avoided. Agave, maple syrup, and palm sugar are also ingredients to watch out for.

*Alcoholic Beverages*

Most alcoholic beverages contain plenty of sugar. Mixed drinks, spiked punch, craft beer, or any beverage where fruit juice and other mixers are added to the sugar content are the main offenders. But most types of alcohol are sugar- and carb-heavy before anything else is even added. Wine is very high in carbs and sugar because it is made with fermented grapes, and grapes themselves have a high sugar content. Beer is brewed from grains like barley and wheat, which makes most beer high in carbohydrates.

If you want to drink without all of the sugar, choose options that are low in calories, carbs, and sugars. Whiskey and brandy tend to have no carbs, as does tequila and unflavored vodka. Just be sure to avoid flavored versions which increase the carb count.

Too much alcohol can also generally harm your body, especially your liver, and like sugar, alcohol can be an unhealthy way to manage your emotions without dealing with the problems that caused the emotions in the first place. Restrict alcoholic beverages to only occasional consumption to avoid both the sugar risks and the other unfortunate side effects of drinking too much alcohol on a routine basis.

## THE IMPORTANCE OF READING LABELS

How do you know how much sugar content something has? If you're uncertain and you need to double check, just read the nutrition label. Many people skip over these labels when they're deciding what they want from the grocery store, but they contain plenty of important information that can keep you from cheating on your sugar detox, accidentally or purposefully. Make reading the labels on the food you buy part of your grocery store routine so you can be certain that everything you bring back home with you is sugar detox compliant.

Start with the nutrition facts on the packaging, specifically the carbohydrate count. Food with high carbs typically means that item will be packed with sugar. But weigh that number against the fiber count, and subtract the grams of fiber from the total number of carbs. Your body cannot digest fiber in the same way it can break down both simple and complex sugars, so it does not pose as much of a risk to your blood sugar levels or overall health. But remember that a high fiber count does not make up for any other sugars the product might contain. Something that has 32 grams of carbs, 10 of which are fiber, still has 22 grams of carbs that will affect your body's blood sugar and can contribute to health problems.

Next, take a look at the ingredient list. Keep an eye out for any mention of sugar or other sweeteners like honey and corn syrup. Also look for other words for sugar that hide its presence in the item, such as fructose, glucose, dextrose, maltose, and sucrose. These are all types of sugar in different forms, and though they may not sound like it at first glance, sugar by any other name would taste just as sweet—and be just as damaging to your health.

Not everything you see in the grocery store has a nutrition label readily available. Produce is often unlabeled, even though many fruits are high in sugar. Reading the label is a helpful step, but it is not the be-all-end-all of learning which foods are good for you and which will introduce tons of sugar into your diet. When in doubt, you can use certain websites and apps for nutritional information on unlabeled foods, which we will discuss in more detail later.

*What's Left?*

After throwing so many things out of your pantry and fridge, you may be wondering what's left for you to eat. It can seem like you've thrown half your kitchen out and you hardly have enough available to make a decent meal. The good news is that despite how many foods contain sugar, there are still plenty of options left for meals that have little to no sugar content. Diet staples like most vegetables, meat and other proteins, and healthy carbs like whole grains, are still on the table and are more than enough to make a delicious meal out of. Eating sugar tends to lock us into the habit of eating the same few foods every week. Mix up the ingredients you use to break that repetitive cycle and make dinner exciting again. You just might expand your food horizons and find dishes you've never tried before that end up becoming your new favorites.

3

## STEP 2

MAKE HEALTHY REPLACEMENTS

Now you know what kinds of foods you should get rid of. The next step is to identify and stock up on the foods that assist your sugar detox. While it may seem that a large portion of your typical trip to the grocery store has just been eliminated from your shopping cart, there are still many excellent, low-sugar foods available. If your diet is restricted by food allergies or the decision to eat a certain way—for example, vegan and vegetarian diets—rest assured that there are options in all different areas of the food pyramid that can fit any diet or lifestyle.

It is important to replace foods in your diet with healthy alternatives rather than just cutting them out. When trying to quit any bad and addictive habit, replacing it with a good habit is much easier than just trying to end an existing habit. This is the same reason why people trying to quit smoking will chew gum whenever they get the urge to smoke. Replacement behaviors give your brain and your body something else to occupy them. Without this replacement, you have nothing to think about other than the habit you are trying to quit, and thinking about it for extended periods of time can make you more likely to cave. Instead, you can focus on building a new habit, which keeps you from ruminating on what you aren't allowing yourself to do.

You may find a whole new menu full of breakfast, lunch, and dinner staples you've never tried before, or you may only need to make small adjustments to swap out ingredients that are high in sugar. For sugary foods that you crave frequently, you may want to have a specific replacement you indulge in every time you get the craving for that food. For example, if you typically open a can of soda when you are feeling stressed or tired, replace it with something similar enough to fulfill the urge but different enough that it is a healthy alternative. You might try sugar-free seltzer or a carbonated water like Perrier. If you tend to snack on something crunchy like trail mix, try carrot and celery sticks for all of the crunch with none of the added sugar. These replacements work best when they are foods you enjoy, so find something that tastes good enough that you don't really miss the food you were originally craving.

## FOODS YOU CAN STILL EAT

Once you've gotten rid of everything you aren't allowing yourself to have, fill your kitchen and pantry back up with these healthier options. Give yourself plenty to choose from so you can find a replacement meal for all manners of cravings. If you're open to it, now is a great time to try out some new dishes and ingredients that you've never used before. This can help make your eating habits more varied and get you excited about starting a new diet. It's easy to get discouraged by all the things you aren't allowed to eat anymore, so focus instead on all of the new options available to you. You will see just how much variety and novelty you can still have in your diet.

*Meat*

Protein is incredibly important during a sugar detox. It helps provide a fairly large portion of your energy when simple carbs are removed from the equation, and it is a great center plate item that is naturally free of sugar. All sources and cuts of meat in their natural, unprocessed form make for great meal options during a sugar detox, and you can eat meat as often as you like without raising your sugar levels.

There are plenty of options when it comes to meat. You can go with traditional staples like chicken, pork, and beef. You can include turkey, lamb, and goat. You may even have access to more uncommon choices like bison and venison. Dark and white meat alike are both acceptable options.

The only thing you should watch out for are meats that have been heavily processed and may have had sugar added to them in a sauce or marinade. Pork ribs, for example, often come served with sauce, but even before that they are frequently marinated with sugary ingredients. Other processed meats like bacon, ham, sausage, and salami carry this danger as well, so be wary and check the packaging for nutrition information to be sure that hidden sugars are not sneaking into your diet.

If you are a vegetarian or vegan, meat is off the menu. However, this does not mean there is no way for you to get your protein while still eating a low-sugar diet. There are many sugar-free sources of protein available to you which we will discuss later on.

*Seafood*

Seafood is another great way to get your protein without needing to worry about sugar. This includes both saltwater and freshwater fish, as well as shellfish. Some people believe there isn't much variety in taste when it comes to fish, but in actuality fish tastes very different depending on the species and the way you prepare it. If you've tried seafood before and it wasn't particularly appealing, try a different type of fish or shellfish and see if that is more to your taste. Sometimes it is only a matter of adding lemon or butter to make seafood one of your new favorites.

There are many types of fish that are commonly available in most areas. Salmon, cod, tuna, herring, and tilapia can be found either frozen or fresh in most stores. Salmon in particular has recently been singled out as a great addition to any diet due to its high Omega-3 content, a fatty acid which supports heart, joint, and brain health. Don't let the "fat" in the name fool you; salmon is a very healthy choice, as are similar fish which are also high in Omega-3. Other fish options to add to your diet include swordfish, catfish, anchovies, flounder, mackerel, halibut, and snapper.

Shellfish is just as good to add to your diet as fish. Grill or pan fry some shrimp, or steam some clams or mussels. Include some crab and lobster in your diet, so long as you don't break the bank. Scallops and oysters make for good choices as well. All of these are foods you can eat completely guilt-free on a sugar detox cleanse.

*Most Vegetables*

The vast majority of vegetables are very low in sugars and carbs, which means they can be safely consumed on a low sugar diet. Vegetables contain plenty of vitamins and minerals that are important for a balanced diet, so make sure to include plenty of them in your meals and snacks. You can have everything from broccoli to green beans to bell peppers. Leafy greens are a great choice, especially nutrient-dense choices like kale and spinach. Cauliflower and zucchini are especially popular choices for low-sugar and low-carb diets due to their versatility in sugarless replacements for high-carb foods like zucchini spaghetti and cauliflower rice.

If you're someone who had trouble finishing their veggies as a kid and hasn't grown into the habit of eating them as an adult, mixing up the way you prepare your vegetables can make eating them much more palatable. Roasting, pan frying, and grilling can improve the flavor of most vegetables, as can the right sugar-free seasoning or sauce. With the right cooking method, veggies can go from a necessity to a delicious part of every meal.

WHILE MOST VEGETABLES are fine to eat on a sugar detox, there are a few you should avoid. Root vegetables like potatoes can be a problem if you eat too many. They are packed with carbs, which raises your blood sugar level with minimal health benefits. Eat them sparingly if at all.

*Some Fruits*

Many fruits are very high in sugar, which automatically puts them on the list of foods to avoid. However, this isn't true for every fruit. In fact, some fruits are actually surprisingly low in sugar and can be consumed in low to moderate amounts. The difference between acceptable and unacceptable fruits lies in their glycemic index.

The glycemic index of a food is a measure of the impact it has on your blood sugar. Some foods raise your blood sugar very quickly, while others raise your blood sugar slower for a longer lasting energy boost. For carb-heavy foods, "Foods low on the glycemic index (GI) scale tend to release glucose slowly and steadily," while "Foods high on the glycemic index release glucose rapidly" (Harvard Health Publishing, 2020, para. 1). High GI foods give you that sharp energy boost and drop off commonly related to sugary foods. Low GI foods, on the other hand, do not have as strong of an effect on your blood sugar or your mood, so they are much safer to eat on a sugar detox diet.

Fruits with a low GI are okay to eat on your diet. These include grapefruit, pears, cherries, peaches, apricots, and kiwis, to name a few. Many kinds of berries like raspberries and blackberries are relatively low in sugar and have a lower GI as well. In general, fruits with a GI below about 50 are safer to consume on a more frequent basis than those with a GI above 50, but the lower the better. Cherries are notably low with an average GI of

22, so they are the best choice if you are looking for a sweet snack that won't set back your progress. Note that other factors can influence the GI of a food. Cooking food tends to raise its GI, and over-ripened fruits have a higher GI than under-ripened fruits of the same kind.

Fruits that have a very high GI can be consumed, but only on a very occasional basis. Don't overload on these kinds of fruits or you will undo all of the hard work you are putting in. Fruits to limit your consumption of or avoid entirely include pineapple, watermelon, and dates. Even if a fruit has a low GI, you should still limit how often it occurs in your diet to avoid raising your blood sugar levels, but occasional pieces of fruit are okay.

*Nuts & Seeds*

Nuts and seeds are very low in sugar and don't have much impact on your glucose levels. A handful of almonds, cashews, pecans, pine nuts, or sunflower seeds makes for a great snack. Many nuts and seeds are used in cooking, such as sesame seeds and walnuts, and they can be incorporated into a number of different dishes to add extra flavor and texture.

One word of caution when it comes to nuts is that you should avoid most flavored nuts and go for plain or lightly salted instead. Honey roasted nuts may taste a bit better than the regular version, but the addition of honey and other additives means they are high in sugar as well, making them a less healthy choice. Skip trail mix as well, as it often includes dried fruit and pieces of chocolate or other candy that detracts from the healthiness of the snack.

*Legumes & Beans*

Legumes and beans are another great choice to keep on hand. They may be a bit higher in carbs than other options, but they are also high in fiber and very low in sugar. There are plenty of options to choose from, each of which can be used in a number of different ways. Chickpeas can be cooked on their own or mashed up to make hummus. Black beans make as good a soup as they do a side dish, and they are commonly featured in Mexican cuisine. So are refried beans, which are most commonly made with pinto beans. Other good options include peas, red beans, kidney beans, black eyed peas, lentils, and lima beans.

*Whole grains*

Many people believe that cutting sugar means cutting all carbs, but this does not have to be the case. It's true that on a sugar detox cleanse you don't want to eat a lot of white bread or white rice because they are made of refined carbs, which makes them high in sugar. However, this does not mean that carbohydrates like rice and bread are completely off the table. Carbs are still very important to your body's functions, even if some are less good for you than others. The key is choosing healthy carbs and cutting unhealthy ones. You just need to make sure you are eating non-refined versions of these foods to avoid the addition of sugar. You can do this by sticking to whole grain options rather than those made with white flour.

Whole grains are made with complex carbohydrates rather than simple carbs. This makes them better options on a sugar detox diet. Similar to low GI fruit, whole grains are less likely to cause a spike in your blood sugar. You can eat bread, rice, some cereals and oatmeals, and some pasta so long as you choose products that are made with whole grains. These grains include whole grain oats, barley, quinoa, amaranth, brown rice, millet, rye, and buckwheat among many others. If you consistently choose carb sources that are full of whole grains and make sure to always check the packaging of any bread or wheat item to confirm its ingredients, you can skip the hidden sugar that is so commonly found in many bread products.

*Eggs and Dairy*

Eggs and dairy products are a good option for incorporating protein into your diet and for adding some variety to low-sugar meals. Instead of a bowl of cereal for breakfast, eggs are a great way to start your day. Pair this with a glass of milk for a healthy and sugar-free breakfast—though you should be careful of potential added sugars in 1% or fat-free milk. Many dairy products can be used in cooking in surprisingly inventive ways. For example, if you're making a casserole but you want to skip the breadcrumbs or puff pastry that would otherwise result in a sugary dish, you can mix in some cream cheese to give the casserole stability without it having a bready top and bottom. And of course, cheese goes great with everything.

When you buy dairy products, make sure you get the unsweetened versions. This means plain yogurt, unsweetened butter, plain cream cheese, and similar options. Dairy may be on the menu, but sugary flavorings, sweetened coffee creamers, and ice cream are not. Make the smart choice and always check how many grams of sugar something contains before adding it to your cart.

You can also use dairy replacements if you are lactose intolerant or if you want to further reduce your sugar intake. Go for unsweetened coconut milk, almond milk, or soy milk for naturally lactose-free and sugar-free options. You can also buy "dairy" products made with these milk replacements such as nut-based cream cheese and yogurt.

### ADDING SOME SWEETNESS BACK INTO YOUR DIET

Many sources of sweetness are restricted or banned on a sugar-free diet. You cannot have many sweet treats like candy, cookies, or cake. Foods that use sweeteners such as honey and corn syrup will raise your blood sugar just as quickly as regular sugar, if not more so. Refined carbs aren't particularly sweet, but even they pose a danger to your success in transitioning to a sugarless lifestyle. Even natural sources of sugar like many fruits and some vegetables are off-limits. With so many sugary foods off the table, what do you do when your body is desperate for something sweet?

You have to get rid of many sugary products on a sugar detox, but, contrary to popular belief, you don't have to completely eliminate sweetness from your diet. There are still many ways that you can satisfy your sweet tooth and calm your taste buds. We have already discussed some acceptable natural sources of sugar for your body. These include low-GI fruit which can still taste sweet without the negative impact on your body, and whole grain bread products that provide slow, gradually released energy rather than a rapid spike. However, these are not the only ways you can indulge in something sweet. If you are looking for another option, turn to the low- or no-calorie sweeteners that can alter the taste of foods without negatively impacting your blood sugar.

There are many different kinds of sweeteners that are okay to use on a sugarless diet. One notable zero-calorie sweetener is Stevia, which has become fairly popular and accessible recently as the demand for sugar alternatives has increased. It is made from the leaves of the stevia plant. Stevia provides the same sweetness with a much lower risk of high blood sugar, high calorie intake, or other health troubles related to pure sugar. Another option to consider is xylitol, which is a sugar alcohol derived from plants. As a sugar alcohol, it is very sweet but it does not impact your blood sugar. A teaspoon of xylitol also has far fewer calories than a teaspoon of sugar, which can help to control and limit weight gain when snacking on something sweet or improving the flavor of a meal.

Multiple artificial sweeteners contain no calories, though you should still be cautious about how often you consume them. If you aren't careful you may accidentally develop a dependency on these new sweeteners that only worsens your sugar cravings. In general, all things are best in moderation, even when their effect on your blood sugar level is minimal. Still, they are a better choice than indulging in sugary foods, so you can use them as a back-up plan for when your sugar cravings get too strong to ignore.

If these sugar-free sweeteners are allowed, does that mean that you can be on a sugar detox and still have something like diet soda? The answer to this question is a little more complex than it appears on the surface. In one respect, the sweeteners used to make diet soda don't put you in danger of blood glucose level spikes because your body does not metabolize them in the same way as regular sugar sodas. They are a better alternative than just drinking sugary sodas and juices, though "healthier" does not necessarily mean "healthy."

On the other hand, the chemical sweeteners common to soda, though FDA approved, have had some controversy surrounding them for potential negative health effects. Multiple studies have linked both diet and regular soda consumption with type 2 diabetes, with one finding "a significant link between diet soda and the development of high blood sugar levels and body fat, two factors of metabolic syndrome" that could indicate the potential for more serious conditions (Johnson, 2018, para. 12). It should be noted that this does not necessarily prove a strong cause and effect relationship between certain artificial sweeteners and the risk of type 2 diabetes, but it does suggest a relationship of some nature between the two factors.

Ultimately, while these drinks aren't actively harmful to your blood glucose level, they don't do you many favors either. They provide no nutritional value, and since they are diuretics, they don't even hydrate you. On top of that, because they are so sweet, your weakness for sugary drinks may simply switch over to a weakness for diet soda, which still leaves you using food to manage emotional distress and cravings rather than finding a healthier alternative and dealing with these issues in a more organic way. So while diet soda and similarly sweetened products aren't completely off-limits, consuming them in excess goes against the spirit of the sugar detox. You want to make healthier choices, not just choices that appear healthier on the surface but ultimately keep you exactly where you started. You can have sweetened foods and drinks on occasion, but try to keep your choices as healthy as possible and keep your consumption of these artificial sweeteners relatively low for the best results.

## EAT HEALTHY CARBS

As previously mentioned, there is a difference between healthy carbs and unhealthy carbs. There has been a recent tendency with the rise of low-carb diets like the ketogenic diet and the Atkins diet to label all carbs as the same thing and ban them all from your diet, but such a generalization ignores the varying health impacts of different types of carbs. You are not going to experience the same blood sugar impact from a slice of white bread as you would from a slice of whole wheat bread, nor are fries smothered in ketchup comparable to a side of brown rice. This is because whole grains are a type of complex carbohydrates, while many sugars that make up other sources of carbs are simple carbohydrates.

*Complex Vs. Simple Carbohydrates*

Some carbohydrates are simple and others are complex. The difference between the two lies in their chemical structure. All carbohydrates are made up of sugars, but the length and type of those sugars differs. Simple carbohydrates are relatively small structures made up of just a few sugar molecules. Complex carbohydrates are, as the name suggests, long chains of sugar molecules with a more complex structure. The variance in carbohydrate length makes simple carbs easy for your body to digest rapidly, while complex carbs require a bit more work.

The small size of simple carbohydrates means they can be broken down by your body for energy very quickly. If you have a candy bar or a soda, your body experiences the energy boost nearly instantly because it works to break the simple carbs down into their individual sugars incredibly quickly. This is what leads to a "sugar rush" where you feel re-energized and hyped up by eating sugar, but it can also lead to a heavy crash, as your body exhausts its energy supply very quickly. Because the sugar chain was broken down so quickly, your body burns through the energy it gets from the sugars faster than it gets new energy to replace it. You may have noticed that after eating simple carbs such as candy, white bread, or sugary cereal that your energy levels spike and then rapidly decline just as described. Other sources of simple carbs include most desserts, french fries, pasta made with white flour, and white rice.

Carbohydrates that are complex have a much longer chain of sugars making up the molecule, so they take your body more time to digest. You may even feel a bit tired after eating them rather than immediately energized because your body needs to use its own energy to break the complex carbs down into something usable. Because of this, complex carbs provide steady energy rather than an energy spike. They also fuel you for much longer as they are slowly disassembled over time, meaning that new energy is entering your system throughout the longer digestion process. This makes complex carbs a better source of energy for those who have trouble moderating their sugar intake, as you will have a steadier energy flow instead of rapid peaks and valleys. The longer your energy lasts, the less you must eat to stay energized, and the fewer excess calories you will consume as a whole. Additionally, you free yourself from the mood-based dependency that simple carbs can create because you are not getting an immediate boost. This lessens the risk of seeking out sugar every time you are feeling tired or unmotivated.

Look for complex carbs, typically found in whole grain options as well as many vegetables, and try to replace the simple carbs wherever they appear in your diet. This way, you are still supplying your body with the energy it needs without consuming simple sugars that are bad for your health.

*Healthy and Unhealthy Carbs*

The sugar detox does not aim to eliminate all sources of carbohydrates, nor does it suggest that carbohydrates are inherently a bad thing. Though there has been a recent push to denounce all forms of carbs, the truth is that not all carbs are bad. Some carbs are unhealthy, namely those that fall under the simple and refined carb category, but others do help us get the fuel our bodies need to function efficiently. Without carbs, you would have to drastically increase your consumption of another macronutrient to get the same amount of energy, which could easily turn into overeating. Despite recent popular diets, healthy carbs are crucial for our survival, and they can be a worry-free and guilt-free part of your sugar detox.

# 4

## STEP 3

### INCREASE YOUR PROTEIN INTAKE

You've gotten rid of the things you shouldn't be eating and stocked up on the things you should be, but that doesn't mean the planning phase of the sugar detox cleanse is over. If you just cut out sugar and replace it with whatever you feel like eating without regard for adequate nutrition, you may have a hard time staying on the new diet because you are likely to experience sugar withdrawal symptoms. Intense cravings, low energy, and bad moods are all common in mismanaged attempts to remove sugar from your diet. When you are tired, you get irritable, and your sugar cravings return full-force. You need some way to quiet these symptoms, and fast, before they make you give up on your new commitment altogether.

If you're cutting something out of your diet, you want to replace it with something equivalent. When you reduce your sugar, you can also end up reducing your energy if you aren't careful. Most sugary foods only provide a temporary energy boost, true, but if you lose even the brief energy you get from sugary snacks without replenishing your energy in another way, you will find yourself constantly tired and often cranky. Because of this persistent bad mood, you are much more likely to return to sugar, as it gives you a little boost in both mood and energy.

One method for replacing your energy is using complex carbs instead of simple ones as discussed above. While complex carbs are very beneficial, they are not the only nutrient you need, and eating them to the exclusion of other food groups can leave your meal plans lacking, not to mention repetitive. A well-rounded diet is the best approach, so a more optimal strategy involves mixing complex carbs with other food groups that are also low in sugar. This is where protein comes in.

## THE BENEFITS OF PROTEIN

Protein is a very important part of a sugar detox. First and foremost, it is a great source of energy. It takes a bit longer for your body to break down protein than it does carbohydrates, so you can be certain you are getting enough long-term energy throughout the day. Sugar withdrawal can make you tired and jittery, but protein works against these symptoms.

Additionally, protein helps your body repair its tissues and construct many important molecules that keep you functioning properly. This is important for everyone, but it is especially important when you are exercising. If you are using a sugar detox to help manage your weight or to get fit, you have likely taken up some form of exercise to improve your results. Exercise is great for our minds and bodies, so even if you aren't actively trying to lose weight, it's still a good idea to get up and move for part of the day. Tissue and cell damage caused by workouts is repaired more easily by our bodies when we eat more protein. This means less soreness, which allows someone to work out harder, for longer, and burn more calories.

Finally, the vast majority of protein sources are very low in sugars. The same is true for simple carbs. Of course, this does not mean these things cannot be added to proteins; a burger on a bun and covered in ketchup is going to have more sugar than a plain burger patty on its own. This just means that you should be careful what you put on your food, and watch out for any marinades and sauces that could be used in the preparing or cooking process. So long as you keep added sugar away from your meals, protein provides an amazing energy source that is both tasty and good for you. It is also one that can help ease the symptoms of sugar withdrawal.

*Pushing Back Against Withdrawal Symptoms*

We have already discussed some of the most common and most difficult symptoms of sugar withdrawal. These include irritability, energy dips, intense cravings, and a compulsive desire to eat, even when you are not particularly hungry. Protein works to manage and ease many of these symptoms, which can give your detox attempt a higher chance at being a success. The worst thing you can do at this stage, now that you have already put in so much effort into changing your eating habits, is to give up because the cravings got too strong or because your energy was suffering. Eat more protein to control the negative effects that sugar still has over your body during this detox period.

Perhaps the most frequent reason for abandoning an attempt to leave sugar behind is that persistent craving for sugar once you begin a detox. Remember that sugar is addictive, and your body will want to return to it the second anything goes wrong. Cravings for the thing you quit, whether it is food or something else entirely, are very common when trying to manage an addiction. It is the same craving that makes many recovering alcoholics consider having "just one more glass" and causes many recovering gamblers to make "just one more bet." With sugar, you will want "just one more taste." Cravings can keep you shackled to your sugar burden for far longer than you need to be.

Protein helps you quell those sugar cravings, in part because protein reroutes your brain's dopamine production towards healthier triggers. Studies of the relationship between protein and brain chemistry have found that "adding protein to meals helps curb cravings by increasing levels of the brain's reward hormone, dopamine," which in turn "means the brain is quicker to recognise the high-protein meal as a reward, and will remain 'satisfied' with it for longer than a low-protein meal" (Puscas, 2018, para. 3). Your brain rewards you for making the replacement to a healthier food, which lessens the connection you have made between sugar and positive feelings.

Protein also helps limit cravings by keeping you fuller for longer than most other types of foods, even when the protein holds fewer calories. Your body produces many hormones that create the feelings you recognize as hunger or fullness. The hunger hormone called ghrelin will signal that your stomach is empty and in need of food. Rates of ghrelin are highest when you haven't eaten in a while, and production tends to calm down after you eat. At this point, your body produces another hormone called peptide YY, which lowers your appetite. Protein makes you feel more full because it decreases the production of ghrelin and increases the production of peptide YY. You will still feel hungry, of course, but on a high-protein diet your hunger is less likely to be such a powerful force that it causes you to seek out snacks and pile your plate with food. When you add more protein to your diet, you may find your plate size shrinking as your hunger lessens and your cravings subside.

*Long Term Energy*

Low energy is another hurdle that presents itself after quitting sugar. When your energy is low, you don't feel like doing much of anything other than crawling back into bed and taking a nap. This is more than just a minor annoyance; persistent fatigue can interfere with work, your personal relationships, and your ability to fully enjoy your life. Raising your energy levels will effectively give you more time in the day to do everything you need to do. As you spend less time sleeping, or working so slowly and inefficiently you may as well be sleeping, you will have more time to focus on the task at hand.

Protein is broken down slowly in your body, which means it supplies you with a steadier stream of energy for a longer period of time. Rather than being formed by sugar molecules like in carbohydrates, the building blocks that make up proteins are amino acids. Like complex carbs, proteins contain long chains of these amino acids. But unlike complex carbs, these chains are even longer, are arranged in a more intricate pattern, and have stronger links between the amino acids in the chain. Your body burns more calories during the digestion process of protein than it does when digesting fats and carbs because of how difficult it is to break protein down into its individual amino acids for use. The difficulty of this process means that your body takes a while to extract all the energy it can from foods high in protein, which allows you to receive the energy benefits spread out over a longer period of time. Smaller quantities of food translate into more energy with fewer spikes and dips in your overall energy levels.

## STARTING YOUR DAY RIGHT

Breakfast has been referred to as the "most important meal of the day," and in many ways that idea is true. Breakfast jump-starts your day, giving you the energy you need to fully transition from a resting state into an active one. When we start out energized and well-rested, we are more likely to maintain a positive attitude throughout the day and continue to practice healthy habits. These include taking meals on time; a skipped or delayed breakfast can completely throw off your eating schedule for the rest of the day.

What we eat at breakfast is just as important as if we choose to eat or not. A hasty and not particularly healthy breakfast of a few pieces of toast or a bagel fresh out of the toaster might be a time saver, but it doesn't give you the nutrition you need. Even worse is eating dessert foods for breakfast, such as sweet pastries like muffins and donuts. Starting your day off with sugar only makes it more likely that you will continue to crave sugar throughout the day now that you have activated your sweet tooth. You are also much more likely to experience an energy crash in the afternoon, even if you have a filling and healthy lunch. A well-rounded breakfast contains many important nutrients that help us start our mornings off on the right foot. The vitamins and minerals we get from breakfast foods, especially those that are high in protein, fulfill our body's needs from the get-go and set us up for success throughout the rest of the day.

Breakfast is also very important if you are trying to lose weight. When we rest and do not eat for a few hours, our metabolism enters a sort of hibernation mode. If you don't eat in the morning, your body never leaves this state. It continues to preserve the energy you have stored, which means it doesn't start burning calories as efficiently as it otherwise would. This may mean hunger is postponed, but it also means that you're not actually burning many calories during the first half of your day, even if you are exercising. Eating a proper breakfast awakens your metabolism and kick starts your body processes, triggering them to start using new and stored calories.

For all of these reasons and more, you should incorporate protein into breakfast every morning. Ideally, each day should start with at least 35 grams of protein from any source you like. Protein provides a good source of energy. Because that energy takes a while for your body to digest, your metabolism is awakened and kept active, often all the way through to lunch. Protein-rich foods also contain many vitamins and minerals that are critical to our body's function. Whatever your taste buds are, there is a protein source that meets your needs and fits neatly into a healthy, balanced breakfast.

*High Protein Breakfast Ideas*

If you picture a classic hearty breakfast, you more than likely include eggs somewhere in your mental image. Eggs are a staple of breakfast foods, and for good reason. Eggs are very high in protein and they're a good source of healthy fats, both of which can help satiate hunger later in the day. They are also very easy to make, can be prepared in a variety of ways for every taste, and they don't take very long. In the time it takes to wait for your toast and brew your coffee, you can easily fry up two eggs.

If fried eggs aren't your thing, try hard or soft boiled eggs instead. These are a great option because you can prepare them the night before and enjoy them in the morning without any prep work. Scrambled eggs are another option that can be made very quickly. While omelets are typically seen as a more difficult endeavor, they can be perfected relatively easily. They are also very customizable as you can add all sorts of vegetables and cheeses. You may even choose to double up on protein and include some sliced chicken or beef with your egg dish—but you should avoid overly-processed and fatty proteins like bacon and sausage, even if they are common breakfast items. Adding a slice of whole wheat toast can help round out your meal with complex carbs and no additional saturated fat.

If eggs aren't to your liking, you may find dairy products to be more palatable in the morning. A glass of milk or a similar lactose-free replacement goes well with most any breakfast, including a whole grain cereal with no added sugar. Another good option is a sugar-free yogurt, specifically most Greek yogurts. Greek yogurt is more concentrated, which means it contains more protein. Skip the pre-flavored options and make your own flavoring by adding a small amount of a low GI fruit like cherries or strawberries. Cottage cheese is another potential source of protein at breakfast. Feel free to add some chopped up fruit pieces or top your bowl with nuts for some crunch.

For vegans, eggs and dairy are off the menu, but that doesn't mean there's no way to eat a protein-rich meal in the morning. Smoothies and shakes are an amazingly quick breakfast idea that can still have plenty of protein. Use protein-rich ingredients like unsweetened peanut butter and chia seeds, or make use of protein powder. Protein powder can be a useful supplement if you feel like you are having trouble eating enough protein through natural sources. However, be wary that some protein powders contain additional ingredients and sweeteners that can raise the amount of sugar you're putting in your breakfast. Avoid the more extravagantly flavored powders and stick to more basic flavors, and always check the label before buying and using any protein powder. Another vegan- and vegetarian-compliant option for a high-protein breakfast is avocados. Avocados can be spread on whole grain toast, blended into a creamy green smoothie, or simply enjoyed on their own with a pinch of salt. The options for protein at breakfast are endless, so there are plenty of opportunities to make sure you start your day off with a filling and healthy meal.

## PROTEIN THROUGHOUT THE DAY

Of course, breakfast shouldn't be the last time you have protein for the rest of the day. There are opportunities to add some protein into every meal, and when you do, you will experience the same craving-reducing and energy-boosting benefits you get from a protein packed breakfast.

The best way to ensure that you are getting enough protein in your diet is to include at least one high quality source of protein in every meal. You can have some lean chicken breast cut up and added to a salad, or you can make yourself a side of quinoa to go with your dinner. Have some hummus as a small snack between meals, or bring a cup of yogurt with you to work. As long as you include some protein in every meal, you are unlikely to feel that your cravings are unsatisfied, and less likely to miss sugar very much at all.

In general, you should try to stick to leaner cuts of meat and other low-fat protein options. Some fat is okay and necessary for the proper functioning of your body's systems, but you don't want to overload yourself. When you do include fat in your diet, it is better to eat monounsaturated and polyunsaturated fats than saturated and trans fats. This means choosing healthy oils, nuts, and fish over fried foods, high fat cuts of red meat, coffee creamer, and various snack foods.

*Non-Meat Sources of Protein*

We have already discussed some of the meatless options for protein at breakfast. There are many more options you can use to fulfill your protein needs at lunch and dinner. Plants provide a great deal of protein without sugar so long as you go for whole ingredients rather than pre-made and prepared foods. For example, vegan cream cheeses are often fairly high in protein, but they tend to contain added sugars as well. You are better off using naturally vegan and vegetarian foods rather than plant-based versions of animal products to minimize the chances of added sugar in your diet.

Luckily, there are many various protein sources that are readily available to you. Beans are an amazing meatless source of protein, and they can be combined with brown rice or quinoa for a protein-packed simple lunch or dinner. Lentils are another good source of protein, as are chickpeas and tofu. All of these options naturally contain low or no sugar, and they can all be used to make delicious, filling meals for lunch and dinner.

## HIGH PROTEIN FOODS

Protein is found in so many different kinds of foods. When looking for high protein foods without sugar, there are some more obvious options such as meat and some less obvious choices like nuts and oats. What you choose to include in your diet is up to your own personal tastes and your dietary restrictions, but there is a way to include a healthy amount of protein in every meal no matter how narrow your food options are. To keep meal times interesting, try to rotate what food you're using to get your protein throughout the day, and make different meals each week. Variety will keep dinnertime fun and interesting rather than repetitive, which increases your chances of successfully sticking to your diet.

*Meat and Poultry*

When most people think of protein, they probably picture meat first and foremost. Meat is an amazing source of protein that is naturally varied. If you don't want to include too much red meat in your diet, go for chicken instead. If poultry's not your thing, try pork or something more unusual like venison or bison. Turkey is another great option that has the added benefit of being a naturally lean meat. As previously mentioned, the only meat you should avoid completely is overly processed meats that contain high amounts of sugar in the marinating, curing, and flavoring process. This means most hams, ribs, bacon, and similar foods.

When choosing what type of meat to pick up at the grocery store, you should stick to lean cuts more often than fattier cuts. This means choosing chicken and turkey more frequently than you choose burger patties and steaks. You can have these fattier meats in moderation, but it is better for your overall health to make them an occasional indulgence rather than giving them a starring role on your meal plan, even if there is no sugar added either way. You want to make healthy choices in general, not just sugar-free ones.

*Fish*

If chicken just isn't cutting it for you, turn to fish for a meal with plenty of flavor even without seasoning. Fish are full of protein and healthy fats like Omega-3 fatty acids that keep you feeling fuller for longer. They also provide many important nutrients that your body cannot function without. One of the best fish to start including in your diet is salmon. Salmon has recently been labeled a "superfood" by many people, and this is not without reason. It is full of antioxidants, vitamin B12, and potassium. It is a great protein source that doesn't have the same saturated fat content as red meat. The Omega-3 fatty acids contained in salmon support both your brain and your heart, leading many to call salmon a "brain food" as well. You can't go wrong by adding it to your weekly meals.

If salmon isn't to your taste, or if you'd just like to vary up your fish options, there are many other fish options that have high amounts of protein. Tuna is incredibly high in protein and can be easily turned into a meal for any time of day. Mix it with some low sugar mayonnaise for a quick tuna salad that you can spread on whole wheat bread for a sandwich, or mix tuna salad with lettuce and fresh veggies for a lower carb option. Anchovies, trout, snapper, cod, halibut, and flounders are all high-protein fish that can either be eaten as a center plate item or used to bring more flavor and nutrition to a recipe. Just about any fish is a good choice, so try a few different kinds and see what you like best.

*Shrimp*

Fish isn't the only seafood that's full of protein. Shellfish, specifically shrimp, are also very high in nutrients. Shrimp contain antioxidants and Omega-3 fatty acids just like salmon. They also have vitamins and minerals including iodine, selenium, vitamin B12, phosphorus, and iron. Alongside all of these great attributes, shrimp is also a very low calorie food that is still fairly filling due to its protein content. You can generally consume shrimp guilt-free without needing to keep careful track of your calories because they are unlikely to lead to a caloric imbalance.

In addition to their health benefits, shrimp are an especially flexible ingredient for meals. You can of course enjoy shrimp on their own with a little bit of butter, lemon, or a low-sugar cocktail sauce. Alternatively, you can use them as an ingredient in a variety of recipes. Shrimp scampi is a great option as long as you use whole wheat pasta. Shrimp also pairs nicely with fruits and vegetables like spinach and tomatoes. Coconut shrimp is another great idea, since shredded coconut is relatively low in sugar. Shrimp can be pan-fried, grilled, or baked—just avoid breading it, as most breadcrumbs are made with refined white flour. Season shrimp with lemon and garlic in most circumstances and you are all set to have an amazing meal.

Wild-caught shrimp is viewed as a bit healthier than farm-raised shrimp due to the potential for higher rates of mercury in the farm-raised option, but the risk of negative effects from mercury is very low unless you are eating shrimp for every single meal each day. Typically, you can eat whichever variety is available without too high of a risk of negative effects.

*Eggs*

As mentioned previously, eggs are a great way to get some protein into your breakfast. Their ability to be cooked in a variety of ways means you can have eggs fairly frequently without overdoing it. It also means that they are good for more than just breakfast. Hard boiled eggs can become snacks with just a sprinkle of salt, or perhaps a little avocado and some hot sauce if you enjoy spice. They can also be turned into deviled eggs with minimal work, or sliced up and added to a salad. Fried eggs can be incorporated into a brown rice and lentil bowl as a low-sugar alternative to a ramen bowl. Frittatas and quiches are great choices for any time of day. You can even make scrambled egg tacos. When it comes to eggs, your options are practically limitless for this incredibly versatile food.

*Nuts*

Nuts are a great snack in between meals. They can tide you over between breakfast and lunch if your energy is running low, or get you through to the end of the day at work before dinner. Nuts are very easy to take with you and don't require any prep work or refrigeration, making them a convenient protein option for any time of day.

Nuts can also be included in many recipes. Cashew or peanut chicken works great with a sugar-free peanut or soy sauce. Nuts are a good topping on salads and on different kinds of finger foods. Pine nuts in particular are packed with flavor and healthy fats, and go great with all kinds of dishes. They can add crunch and flavor to a pasta sauce like pesto, which skips the sugar in favor of nuts and herbs.

*Oats*

Oats are very low in sugar and high in protein. Oatmeal isn't something you think of when you're trying to get a lot of protein, but it can be a great meal on a sugar detox that doesn't take very long to make at all. You can also use oats in other meals like overnight oat jars and a sugar-free granola replacement.

The only thing you should watch out for when eating oats are additives that could make the meal more sugary. Many boxed oatmeals are flavored with cinnamon sugar, artificial fruits, and other unhealthy additions. You are better off getting plain oats and making your own oatmeal, only adding in what you want and keeping the sugar count low.

*Cottage Cheese*

The primary protein in cottage cheese is called casein. It takes your body a bit longer to digest casein than other proteins, which makes it a better protein source for long lasting energy. It is also better at supporting muscle strength and preventing the breakdown of muscle tissues after exercise. For these reasons, cottage cheese is an incredible protein source for maintaining energy in an active lifestyle.

There have been many recent recommendations by dieticians and nutritionists to eat a few spoonfuls of cottage cheese before bed. This is because of the casein protein. If we don't eat anything before bed, our metabolisms slow nearly to a halt; on the other hand, if you eat something sugary before bed, your body metabolizes it too quickly and you can find it hard to fall asleep. Casein-heavy cottage cheese is the perfect compromise between these two extremes. As your body slowly breaks down the protein throughout the night, your metabolism remains active, which lets you burn fat even while you are fast asleep.

Cottage cheese is commonly enjoyed as a snack on its own just fine, but you can mix it up a bit if you start getting bored of it. Slice up some fruit with a low GI, and sprinkle just a pinch of cinnamon—not cinnamon sugar—on top. Alternatively, you can use it as a dip for low-sugar vegetable slices. If you're not a huge fan of the chunkier texture of cottage cheese, you can blend it for a few seconds to make it creamier and more palatable.

*Yogurt and Milk*

Yogurt is another dairy product that is high in protein and low in sugar. People who regularly include yogurt in their diet experience, on average, higher energy levels and fewer problems with irregular and upset stomachs. This is because yogurt is also a great source of probiotics. These are good bacteria that live in your gut and keep your digestive system regular. Probiotics also exist in pill and gummy supplement form, but it is much easier and tastier to include some yogurt in your diet. The best kind of yogurt for protein is Greek yogurt. Greek yogurt has a higher concentration of casein compared to whey and provides more protein to your body in general.

Regular milk is a good source of protein as well. Milk

contains both casein and whey proteins. It has many other benefits that make it worthy of inclusion in your diet. The calcium in milk keeps your bones strong, which helps you resist injuries and avoid conditions like osteoporosis as you age. Another benefit of milk is its potassium, which supports a healthy blood pressure, and vitamin D, which also aids bone health. If you aren't a huge fan of milk on its own, it is used in many recipes, so there are plenty of opportunities to add dairy protein into your diet.

The only thing to watch out for in regards to milk and other dairy products is how much sugar you are consuming. Lactose is a sugar, albeit a naturally occurring one, and it can influence your blood glucose levels. However, it has a relatively low GI and it is unlikely to cause your blood sugar to spike like candy or desserts would, so you are fine to have milk so long as you do not go overboard.

*Quinoa*

Quinoa is a plant-based protein powerhouse. It is generally considered to be one of the best sources of protein out of all the grains, and for good reason. Just one cup of cooked quinoa can put a significant dent in your protein goals for the day. It contains all nine necessary amino acids that we must get from food and cannot make ourselves. It's a good idea to add a scoop of quinoa to your daily meals as often as possible.

Quinoa makes an amazing replacement for white rice as a side dish. You get all the benefits of the extra protein with none of the sugar. Add a protein and some veggies for a quinoa bowl, or flavor it with garlic, diced vegetables, and a little butter and enjoy it on its own. You can also use quinoa as a protein in your salad or add it to various soups and stews. As a tip, always rinse quinoa before cooking, and cook quinoa in a low-sugar vegetable or chicken broth instead of just water to give it some extra flavor.

*Lentils*

Lentils are a type of legume, just like peas and beans. If you're not familiar with lentils, they can be a bit intimidating to cook because they aren't a common ingredient in most American households, but their protein count makes them well worth adding to your diet. They are a great ingredient in soups, go well with salad, and star in dal, a type of Indian stew.

One important note regarding lentils is that they should never be eaten raw. Raw lentils can be toxic and will likely make you sick, but the toxin in them breaks down during the cooking process so you can enjoy them safely.

*Beans and Seeds*

Beans are one of the most common non-meat sources of protein. They come in many varieties, each with their own unique flavor and uses. Beans are also very high in fiber, which is imperative in a healthy digestive system and helps to reduce their carbohydrate impact.

Seeds are an equally good choice. Chia seeds, sesame seeds, and sunflower seeds are great additions to your diet. Many people include chia seeds in their smoothies, and lightly toasted sesame seeds are involved in many Asian cuisine dishes. Pumpkin seeds are another good choice. Try roasting them in the oven with a little olive oil and seasoning for an especially tasty and nutritious treat.

*Peas*

You may not think of peas right away when you look for high-protein foods, but they are actually fairly protein dense. Like other legumes, peas have minimal naturally occurring sugars and plenty of protein. They are also low in sodium, low in calories, and free of cholesterol and fat, making them an all-around healthy food. Peas make a good side dish to any meal. They can also be combined with other diced vegetables, fresh or frozen, and used as ingredients in meals like stews and casseroles.

*Edamame*

Edamame are a version of soybeans that involves picking them before they have fully ripened. Like any soy product, they provide a good source of protein, as well as a decent amount of vitamin K, antioxidants, and fiber. Some have claimed that edamame can help lower negative LDL cholesterol levels, (Arnarson, 2017, para. 23). Lower cholesterol can potentially decrease the risk of heart disease and other dangerous conditions.

Edamame are typically sold still inside the pods. Despite this, the pods are not edible, so you should remove them from their casing before eating. Some common uses for edamame include salads, stews, soups, noodle dishes, and on their own as a quick and easy snack.

*Soybeans*

Like their prematurely picked cousins, soybeans are equally high in protein. They also have many of the same benefits, including having an effect on cholesterol levels and being high in antioxidants and fiber. Unlike edamame, soybeans are a little more versatile in terms of what they can be used for when cooking. Soybeans are a common ingredient in plant-based meat and dairy alternatives like soy burgers, soy milk, and soy cheese. Tofu is used in many kinds of dishes as a meat replacement. Contrary to popular thought, tofu isn't reserved just for vegetarians and vegans. Tofu is an excellent way to vary your meals and take a break from potential sources of saturated fats by decreasing your meat consumption.

The only thing you should keep an eye on when consuming soy-based products is any sugars that might have been added to improve the flavor of the food. Remember to check the packaging before putting anything in your cart.

*Chickpeas and Hummus*

Chickpeas are a common protein source in many vegetarian and vegan diets. They are also a good source of vitamins and minerals including manganese, folate, and iron. Chickpeas are high in fiber and relatively low in calories for the energy they provide. Many people add chickpeas to salads or roast them for a side dish. They are especially common in Greek dishes like falafel.

Of course, chickpeas are perhaps more popularly known and consumed as hummus. Hummus is made with mashed chickpeas and tahini, a paste derived from sesame seeds. If you are buying pre-made hummus at the store, watch out for any flavorings that might increase the sugar content. If you want to avoid this risk, make your own hummus at home and add only what you like and what fits your diet. Instead of chips and crackers, dip vegetables in hummus for a low sugar option.

*Broccoli and Brussels Sprouts*

You might not think these leafy greens are especially high in protein, but in truth broccoli and Brussels sprouts can be decent protein sources. They are less impressive than center plate items like meat and yogurt, but adding a side of either of these veggies to your meal can raise its overall protein content. On top of that, there are many other reasons to eat both broccoli and Brussels sprouts. Broccoli is especially high in vitamin C, which supports the health of your body tissues. It contains vitamin A and calcium and makes a good alternative to milk in regards to those vitamins. Brussels sprouts are chock-full of various vitamins and minerals, and they're well worth eating. You may have had bad experiences with them as a kid, but just try pan-frying them until they're real crispy. Then use a liberal amount of garlic and you are certain to put your days of hating Brussels sprouts behind you.

## KEEP TRACK OF YOUR PROTEIN CONSUMPTION

It's not always easy to make sure you're getting enough protein in your diet. Even with so many options to choose from, there is still a chance that you will overestimate how much protein is in your meals and fall below your protein goals. Failing to eat enough protein commonly leads to irritability, low energy, more intense cravings for sugar, and a higher chance of giving in to those cravings. Be sure to eat enough protein to avoid these withdrawal symptoms.

You can keep track of your protein consumption in a few different ways. One method is to do it manually with a food journal. With this method, you write out what you eat for each meal and make a note of its nutritional info. You can track calories, protein, carbs, sugars, and anything else you want to keep an eye on like sodium levels and cholesterol. However, you do have to look up and accurately record the nutrition information yourself, which can be a bit of a chore if you're trying to quickly eat and start your next task.

Another option is using websites and apps to help track your eating habits. With these applications, you typically only have to choose the type and amount of food you ate and information about protein, calories, and other nutrition facts will auto populate. These kinds of apps also often let you set goals for certain macronutrients, so you can specify the protein goal you want to hit by the end of the day or for each meal and adjust your meals accordingly. One such app that helps you see the nutritional breakdown of your meals is Cronometer. This app allows you to input your food choices, keep track of how many calories you have burned versus how many you have consumed, and see the breakdown of protein, carbs, and fat that goes into your diet. These can be very helpful tools when trying to limit your sugar and increase your protein, so be sure to make use of all tools available to you.

*Enjoying, Not Obsessing*

While tracking your meals is a good idea, this is only true as long as you refrain from obsessing over what you are eating. You should practice good nutrition, but not at the risk of your mental health or developing a harmful relationship with food.

After all, food is an inherently enjoyable part of your day. It should not become something you dread or spend a large portion of your day stressing over. While you should exhibit some control over what you eat in the sense that you do not want to consume things that are bad for you, rigidly controlling your meals and their contents to the point of obsession is more common in disordered eating than it is in true healthy eating.

If you have a background of disordered eating habits such as anorexia, bulimia, or binging, or you believe you are at a high risk for developing these conditions, you should be wary about how thoroughly you track your macronutrients and calories. Turning eating into a numbers game has the potential to trigger these conditions as it can encourage some people to harm themselves through incredibly restrictive eating habits and feel intense guilt if they miss their mark. Some will also find that tracking protein through these methods is not a good fit for them for other reasons, such as a busy schedule or an inability to remember to enter data. Whatever the reason, the good news is that while apps like Cronometer can be helpful, they are not mandatory to achieve your goal of cutting back on sugar.

It is completely possible to be successful on the sugar detox cleanse without needing to track your protein or constantly critique what and how much you are eating, so there is no need to engage in these strategies if you feel they may be triggers for you. Instead, just focus on eliminating sugary foods and increasing proteins in a more general sense. Do your best to stay healthy both physically and mentally, and don't put one at risk to improve the other. Your whole system, body and mind, needs to be considered when improving your well-being.

*Using Pre-made Meal Plans*

If you believe Cronometer and similar apps could trigger disordered eating symptoms, or if you are having trouble sticking to tracking your protein, another method you can try is making use of meal plans. Meal plans give you a guiding hand when first starting a diet by showing you the kinds of foods that are acceptable and the kinds that should be avoided. They give you a good idea of the balance you should have between proteins, carbs, and fats in your diet. Pre-made meal plans take away the tendency for obsession that can occur with meal tracking because they provide you with the foods and recipes you need without requiring you to do the math on everything you eat. All of the work is done for you, and you can focus on making amazing food that is good for you. The following chapter contains a meal plan for your first week on the sugar detox which can be a good place to start if you are uncertain how to begin.

As you progress further into the diet, you can decide whether you want to keep using meal plans or if you feel you have gotten a good sense for the eating habits that are expected of you. If you decide the latter, you can slowly transition to making your own meal plans or eating more intuitively while still sticking to a low-sugar, high-protein diet.

5

## STEP 4 - WEEK 1

## DO MORE THROUGH MEAL PLANNING

When starting a new diet, it is important to take the guesswork out of the equation. You want a strong start, and that means avoiding any slip-ups in the first few days. It is easy to misunderstand the requirements of a diet or to forget which foods aren't allowed to be eaten, especially if the diet is a drastic change from what you are used to. This is very likely true for you if you are starting a sugar detox cleanse, as previously sugar may have seemed to dominate the vast majority of your meals, whether you realized it at the time or not. With a meal plan, the road ahead of you will be clear, your weekly goals will be well defined, and the steps you need to take to reach those goals should be evident.

A week one meal plan helps you accomplish all this and more. By learning the types of ingredients and meals that are acceptable on a low-sugar diet, you can more easily incorporate these kinds of foods into your diet. Even if you don't like every meal, you can choose those you like and find substitutions for those you don't. Following a meal plan takes some of the hassle and confusion out of starting a diet by telling you exactly what you need to eat every day. It ensures that you are starting off on the right foot and following the trajectory that will allow you to keep practicing good eating habits.

The week one meal plan also gives you guidance on how you should plan your grocery trips in the future. It is a good idea to do some meal planning of your own once you hit the end of week one. Come up with a series of dishes you want to make throughout the week that sound tasty and also fulfill your nutrient needs. List these ingredients on paper or on your phone, and then head to the grocery store and buy only what you need. This process limits unnecessary and impulse purchases at the store which may not be sugar detox compliant and encourages you to make smart choices. If you have an especially busy weekday, meal planning eliminates the time you would otherwise spend trying to come up with what to make for dinner each night and ensures that your meals throughout the week are varied enough to stay interesting and keep you on your diet.

STARTING YOUR DETOX

How do you go about starting a sugar detox? Is it a gradual shift from sugary foods that eventually ends in minimizing sugar in your diet, or is it better to start off by eliminating all problematic foods at once? The sugar detox suggests following the latter format, as this gets you into the right mindset for avoiding sugars more rapidly and reduces the risk of cravings after the first few weeks which might otherwise linger if you allowed yourself higher amounts of sugar.

Start off your first week by doing your best to cut out all forms of carbs, both simple and complex. Obtain your energy primarily from protein, and avoid foods high in sugars and grains. Continue this behavior for the first three days. After this pattern has been established, you can slowly start loosening the restrictions. On day four, some healthy sources of carbs are okay, such as fruit with a low GI that won't impact your blood sugar much. Later in the week, you can reintroduce whole grains and zero-calorie sugar alternatives like Stevia. This ensures you will not run out of energy, but also teaches you that you can indeed survive on low to no sugar in your diet.

## CALORIE GUIDELINES

Getting adequate nutrition throughout the week is important, even while you are cutting out certain things from your diet. You should still make sure you are eating enough calories throughout your day to maintain high energy levels and reduce the risk of crashing or caving.

The calories you need are determined by a variety of individual factors, but some general parameters do exist. Assuming moderate physical activity, adult males should try to eat about 2,600 to 3,000 calories a day, while adult females should aim for 1,800 to 2,200 calories. The difference is a result of body composition and nutritional need differentiation between women and men, though these numbers are by no means absolute. The calories children should consume in a day are different based on the child's age. Consult a pediatrician or a nutrition expert for more specific information about what your child needs to stay fit and strong.

## WEEK ONE MEAL PLAN

In week one, you want to follow the basic meal plan outline explained herein. The first few days will be low-to-no carb meals, followed by the gradual increase of carbohydrates. By the end of the week, all foods that are acceptable on a sugar detox will become available to you, but it is important to start out relatively strict to lessen the risk of reverting to your old ways.

*Day One*

On day one, you want to focus on giving yourself enough energy and nutrients throughout the day to support your needs. You are just starting to transition away from sugar, so the cravings should not hit too hard, but the high amounts of protein should help ease any cravings that do occur.

*Breakfast - Green Smoothie*

Green vegetables are a staple of any low-carb diet, and smoothies are a great way to get all the nutrition you need. Add in some avocado and you have a delicious, creamy smoothie that hardly tastes like the start of a diet at all!

**Time:** 5 minutes
**Serving Size:** 1
**Nutritional Facts:**
*Calories:* 452
*Carbs:* 14 g
*Sugar:* 1 g
*Fat:* 17 g
*Protein:* 36 g

**Ingredients:**
- 1 cup unsweetened almond milk
- ½ cup spinach
- ½ avocado
- ⅓ cup unsweetened vanilla protein powder
- 1 tablespoon sugar-free peanut butter

**Directions:**

1. Slice open an avocado and remove the pit. Rinse the spinach.

2. Add almond milk, spinach, ½ of the avocado, protein powder, and peanut butter to a blender. Pulse in 30 second increments until smoothie reaches the desired consistency, or for about one to two minutes.

3. If you want a colder smoothie, use frozen avocado slices, or make the smoothie the night before and leave it in the fridge overnight; re-blending in the morning.

*Snack - Roasted Chickpeas*

THESE ROASTED CHICKPEAS are a great alternative to chips or popcorn. They pack plenty of flavor without any of the added sugar. Eat them on their own or add them to a salad for a tasty crunch.

**Time:** 45 minutes
**Serving Size:** 4
**Nutritional Facts:**
*Calories:* 62
*Carbs:* 5 g
*Sugar:* 1 g
*Fat:* <1 g
*Protein:* 7 g
**Ingredients:**
- 8 oz can of chickpeas
- ½ tbsp olive oil
- ½ tsp garlic powder
- ½ tsp onion powder
- ½ tsp ground cumin
- ½ tsp paprika
- ¼ tsp black pepper

**Directions:**
1. Preheat the oven to 400°F.
2. Rinse chickpeas and dry well. Grease a baking sheet with cooking spray and arrange chickpeas in a single layer. Bake chickpeas in the oven for 15 minutes.
3. While chickpeas are cooking, add olive oil, garlic powder, onion powder, ground cumin, paprika, and black pepper to a bowl. Stir to combine.
4. Remove chickpeas from the oven and transfer to the bowl, coating them in the olive oil and spice mix. Return the chickpeas to the baking sheet and cook for another 20 minutes, stir-

ring once halfway through. Chickpeas should be crispy once done.

*Lunch - Chicken Salad Lettuce Wraps*

With bread off the menu, try lettuce wraps instead. They make a great low-carb alternative and cut out the sugar present in most commercial tortilla wraps.

**Time:** 35 minutes
**Serving Size:** 2
**Nutritional Facts:**
*Calories:* 480
*Carbs:* 4 g
*Sugar:* 2 g
*Fat:* 16 g
*Protein:* 48 g

**Ingredients:**
- ½ lb chicken breast
- 6 romaine lettuce leaves, washed and dried
- 1 cup celery, diced
- ½ cup mayonnaise
- 1 tbsp olive oil
- 1 tsp spicy brown mustard
- ½ teaspoon black pepper
- ½ teaspoon salt

**Directions:**

1. Preheat the oven to 400°F.

2. Add chicken breasts to a large bowl with olive oil, salt, and pepper. Mix to coat and transfer to a lined baking sheet.

3. Roast chicken in the oven for 20-25 minutes. Make sure the interior of the chicken is no longer pink when done.

4. Remove chicken from the oven and let cool. Dice the chicken into ½-inch cubes.

5. Transfer chicken to a bowl. Add celery, mayonnaise, and spicy brown mustard. Mix well.

6. Spoon the chicken mixture into the lettuce leaves and serve.

*Snack - Hard Boiled Eggs*

Hard boiled eggs can be used in a number of ways. You can use them to make deviled eggs, slice them up to top a salad, or just eat them whole with a little salt. Knowing how to make hard boiled eggs ensures you have a relatively quick snack you can make with minimal ingredients.

**Time:** 25 minutes
**Serving Size:** 4
**Nutritional Facts:**
*Calories:* 162
*Carbs:* <1 g
*Sugar:* <1 g
*Fat:* 9 g
*Protein:* 13 g
**Ingredients:**
- 8 eggs
- 1 tsp salt

**Directions:**

1. Place eggs in the bottom of a saucepot. Make sure eggs fit comfortably without overlap.

2. Fill the saucepot with cold water about one or two inches above the eggs. Add salt to the water.

3. Put the pot on the stove and bring to a boil over high heat, uncovered.

4. When the water starts to boil, shut off the heat and cover the pot. Do not remove the pot from the burner. Let eggs sit for 10-12 minutes depending on how firm you want the yolks to be, with a longer cooking time yielding firmer yolks.

5. Transfer eggs to an ice water bath with a slotted spoon. Allow eggs to cool entirely before peeling or storing.

*Dinner - Stuffed Peppers*

Stuffed peppers are a great way to get picky kids to eat their vegetables, but they taste just as great for adults too. To limit the amount of fat in the recipe, ground turkey is used, but you can use a leaner ground beef if you prefer.

**Time:** 50 minutes
**Serving Size:** 4
**Nutritional Facts:**
*Calories:* 470
*Carbs:* 13 g
*Sugar:* 4 g
*Fat:* 20 g
*Protein:* 36 g

**Ingredients:**
- 1 lb ground turkey
- 4 bell peppers
- 1 tomato, diced
- ½ onion, diced
- ½ cup black beans
- ½ cup shredded cheddar cheese
- 1 tbsp hot sauce

**Directions:**

1. Preheat the oven to 400°F.

2. In a skillet on the stove, brown the ground turkey until thoroughly cooked. Add diced onions and cook for an additional five minutes.

3. To the meat mixture, add diced tomatoes, black beans, and cheese. Drizzle on hot sauce and stir.

4. Wash the peppers and cut a circle around the stem to remove the seeds. Cut the peppers lengthwise so each one makes two boats. Scrape any remaining seeds out of the halves.

5. Lay peppers out on a greased baking sheet. Fill with ground turkey mixture and top with any remaining cheese. Transfer peppers to the oven and back for 35-40 minutes, or until peppers are tender and lightly charred on the outside.

*Day Two*

Day two should follow the same pattern that Day One started. Keep sugar and carbs to a minimum, and continue to resist the pull of sugar.

*Breakfast - Egg Stuffed Avocados*

Avocados are an amazing source of healthy fats and protein. They also pair very nicely with eggs. If spice isn't your thing, feel free to leave the hot sauce out and replace it with an extra pinch of salt.

**Time:** 20 minutes
**Serving Size:** 1
**Nutritional Facts:**
*Calories:* 526
*Carbs:* 16 g
*Sugar:* 3 g
*Fat:* 32 g
*Protein:* 34 g

**Ingredients:**
- 2 eggs
- 1 avocado
- ¼ cup cottage cheese
- ½ tsp salt
- ½ tsp black pepper
- ½ tsp hot sauce

**Directions:**

1. Preheat the oven to 400°F.

2. Slice the avocado in half and remove the pit. Crack one egg into the divot left by the pit in each avocado half. Top each with half of the cottage cheese.

3. Put avocado halves on a baking sheet and bake for 15 minutes. Remove from the oven, top with salt, pepper, and a drizzle of hot sauce, and serve.

*Snack - Cold Cut Roll-Ups*

Cold cut roll-ups are pure protein. You can use this recipe as a guideline and substitute any deli meats you like, provided you stay away from over-processed and sweetened cuts.

**Time:** 5 minutes
**Serving Size:** 1
**Nutritional Facts:**
*Calories:* 390
*Carbs:* 4 g
*Sugar:* 2 g
*Fat:* 13 g
*Protein:* 29 g
**Ingredients:**
- ¼ lb turkey, sliced thin
- ⅛ lb cheddar cheese, sliced thin
- 3 romaine lettuce leaves, halved

**Directions:**
1. Lay out turkey slices to make the base of the deli roll-up.
2. Add slices of cheddar cheese and lettuce leaves to each turkey slice. Roll into tube shapes and enjoy.

*Lunch - Lime Grilled Chicken Salad*

USING citrus fruits like lemon and lime let you add flavor to a meal without drastically raising its sugar content. Lime pairs well with chicken breast, so try it out in this lime chicken salad.

**Time:** 20 minutes
**Serving Size:** 2
**Nutritional Facts:**
*Calories:* 491
*Carbs:* 5 g
*Sugar:* 1 g
*Fat:* 13 g
*Protein:* 76 g
**Ingredients:**
- 1 lb chicken breasts

- 1 lime
- ½ avocado, sliced and pitted
- 2 cups romaine lettuce
- ¼ cup cherry tomatoes

**Directions:**

1. Preheat the grill to medium heat. Grill chicken breasts for about 10 minutes depending on their thickness, flipping halfway through.

2. Wait for the chicken to cool, then slice into bite-size strips.

3. Wash and chop lettuce. Top with sliced chicken, avocado, and diced cherry tomatoes. Squeeze lime juice over top and serve.

*Snack - Chia Seed Pudding*

Chia seed pudding is an incredibly easy snack with very few ingredients required. It's great to make in bulk and store in the fridge for an entire weeks' worth of snacks.

**Time:** 5 minutes, refrigerate overnight

**Serving Size:** 4

**Nutritional Facts:**

*Calories:* 131

*Carbs:* 11 g

*Sugar:* 6 g

*Fat:* 7 g

*Protein:* 12 g

**Ingredients:**
- 2 cups unsweetened almond milk
- 8 tbsp chia seeds
- 2 tsp Stevia

**Directions:**

1. Take four mason jars or other resealable containers and fill each with ½ cup almond milk. Mix 2 tablespoons of chia seeds and ½ teaspoon of Stevia into each jar.

2. Seal the jars and allow them to chill for at least two hours,

preferably overnight.

*Dinner - Stir-Fry with Zucchini and Shrimp*

This version of stir-fry doesn't contain a rice base but instead uses zucchini. Later on in the sugar detox diet when healthy carbs are reintroduced, you can repurpose this recipe with brown rice.

**Time:** 20 minutes
**Serving Size:** 4
**Nutritional Facts:**
*Calories:* 203
*Carbs:* 3 g
*Sugar:* 1 g
*Fat:* 9 g
*Protein:* 26 g
**Ingredients:**
- 1 lb shrimp, peeled and deveined
- 1 medium zucchini
- 2 tbsp olive oil
- 2 tbsp garlic, minced
- 1 tbsp ginger
- 1 tsp sesame oil
- 1 tsp sugar-free soy sauce

**Directions:**
1. Wash and slice zucchini into ¼-inch slices.
2. Heat oil in a skillet over medium-high heat. Add shrimp and cook until pink, about two minutes on each side. Remove shrimp from the skillet and set aside.
3. Add zucchini to the skillet and cook until tender, about five minutes. Drain excess water.
4. Return shrimp to the skillet and add garlic, ginger, sesame oil, and soy sauce. Sauté for another five minutes, stirring frequently, and serve.

*Day Three*

There is a good chance your cravings will be especially

tricky to manage as you enter day three. You may be tempted to return to your old eating habits, but stay strong! Add some extra protein into your meals and push back against cravings.

*Breakfast - Simple Scrambled Eggs*

Scrambled eggs are a quick and easy choice for breakfast that give you a great protein start to your day. If you want to add some extra protein to this recipe, cut up and mix in some leftover chicken.

**Time:** 10 minutes
**Serving Size:** 1
**Nutritional Facts:**
*Calories:* 418
*Carbs:* 4 g
*Sugar:* 2 g
*Fat:* 12 g
*Protein:* 44 g

**Ingredients:**
- 2 eggs
- 1 cup plain yogurt
- ¼ cup shredded cheddar cheese
- ½ tbsp butter
- ½ tsp salt
- ¼ tsp black pepper

**Directions:**

1. Crack eggs into a bowl and break yolks with a fork. Add yogurt and beat until frothy.

2. Heat a pan on the stove over medium heat and melt butter. Add egg mixture and stir periodically as eggs firm. Cook for five minutes, and add the shredded cheese when eggs are no longer runny. Sprinkle eggs with salt and pepper.

3. Transfer to a plate and serve.

*Snack - Black Bean Salad*

Black bean salad is a snack option that is both filling enough to keep your energy up in the morning, and also light enough to make for the perfect snack. Mix it up early in the morning and store it in the fridge until lunchtime.

**Time:** 10 minutes
**Serving Size:** 2
**Nutritional Facts:**
*Calories:* 221
*Carbs:* 28 g
*Sugar:* 2 g
*Fat:* 1 g
*Protein:* 13 g
**Ingredients:**
- 1 16 oz can of black beans
- ½ bell pepper
- ½ cup romaine lettuce
- ½ cup cherry tomatoes
- ¼ cup shredded carrot
- 2 tbsp sugar-free vinaigrette (optional)

**Directions:**

1. Empty the can of black beans into a small pot on the stove. Cook on medium heat, stirring occasionally, until beans are tender, about five minutes. Allow beans to cool before proceeding.

2. Chop bell pepper, lettuce, and cherry tomatoes into bite-size pieces. Mix with beans and shredded carrot. Top with vinaigrette and serve or store.

*Lunch - Salmon Fillet*

With the health benefits of salmon, it is a no-brainer food item for a low-carb lunch option. Its bold flavors ensure little work is needed to make this fish stand out.

**Time:** 30 minutes
**Serving Size:** 2
**Nutritional Facts:**
*Calories:* 460
*Carbs:* 2 g

*Sugar:* <1 g
*Fat:* 28 g
*Protein:* 48 g
**Ingredients:**
- 1 lb salmon
- 1 lemon
- 2 tbsp butter
- 1 tbsp garlic, minced
- ½ tsp salt
- ½ tsp black pepper

**Directions:**
1. Preheat the oven to 350°F.
2. Line a baking sheet with aluminum foil. Cut a lemon into thin slices and lay them out, then place the salmon fillet on the slices. Top with melted butter, garlic, salt, and pepper.
3. Fold the foil so it creates a sealed pocket and bake in the oven for 25 minutes. Salmon should be flaky when done.

*Snack - Turmeric Cashews*

Turmeric is a great spice that is both tasty and good for you. It promotes good digestive health and reduces the risk of heartburn, so adding it to roasted cashews is a surefire hit.

**Time:** 25 minutes
**Serving Size:** 2
**Nutritional Facts:**
*Calories:* 130
*Carbs:* 5 g
*Sugar:* 1 g
*Fat:* 7 g
*Protein:* 8 g
**Ingredients:**
- 2 cups raw cashews
- 1 tbsp chia seeds
- 1 tbsp olive oil
- 1 tsp ground turmeric

- ½ tsp salt
- ½ tsp garlic powder

**Directions:**

1. Preheat the oven to 300°F.

2. Add cashew nuts to a bowl along with olive oil, chia seeds, turmeric, salt, and garlic powder. Toss to thoroughly coat the cashews.

3. Spread cashews out on a baking sheet and roast in the oven for 10 minutes. Stir, then return cashews to the oven for another 10 minutes until crispy and golden brown.

*Dinner - Ground Beef and Bean Chili*

Chili is typically a wintertime dish, but this chili tastes good enough you'll find excuses to eat it anytime. Unlike commercially sold chili, this homemade option is very low in sugar.

**Time:** 45 minutes

**Serving Size:** 4

**Nutritional Facts:**

*Calories:* 316

*Carbs:* 34 g

*Sugar:* 2 g

*Fat:* 13 g

*Protein:* 36 g

**Ingredients:**

- 1 lb lean ground beef
- 15 oz can of kidney beans
- 4 tomatoes, diced
- ½ onion, diced
- 1 tbsp garlic, minced
- 1 tbsp olive oil
- 2 tsp chili powder
- 2 tsp ground cumin

**Directions:**

1. In a large pot, add olive oil, beef, onion, chili powder, and

cumin. Brown the beef over medium-high heat, stirring frequently.

2. Add in garlic and tomatoes and cook for five minutes. Pour in two cups of water and let simmer until thickened, about ten minutes. Mix in beans and let them heat through before serving.

*Day Four*

On day four, you can start reintroducing healthy sources of carbs. It's best to start off with natural carb sources. Look for fruits with low sugar levels and low GI. Use these sparingly, but when used well they can really bring some variety to your meals.

*Breakfast - Banana Pancakes*

YOU MIGHT NOT BE able to have the ingredients that go into standard pancake batter, but with a little creativity you can still enjoy pancakes. With the sweetness from bananas, you won't even miss the maple syrup.

**Time:** 15 minutes
**Serving Size:** 4
**Nutritional Facts:**
*Calories:* 233
*Carbs:* 14 g
*Sugar:* 7 g
*Fat:* 3 g
*Protein:* 37 g
**Ingredients:**
- 2 bananas
- 2 eggs
- 1 tbsp protein powder
- 1 tsp butter
- ¼ tsp cinnamon

**Directions:**

1. Peel the bananas and add them to a bowl. Mash them with a fork, then crack eggs into the bowl and add the protein powder. Stir until you have a smooth, slightly runny batter.

2. Heat a griddle or a pan over the stove on medium-high. Grease lightly with butter and let the surface of the pan or griddle get hot before continuing.

3. Pour about two tablespoons of batter into the pan and let it cook for about one to two minutes, waiting until the bottom is relatively firm. Flip with a spatula and let cook for another two minutes, then remove the pancake from the pan.

4. Repeat the previous step until all batter has been used up. Top with cinnamon and serve.

*Snack - Cottage Cheese with Fruit*

Cottage cheese is a perfectly fine snack on its own, but it can be improved with some healthy fruit. This recipe uses cherries as they have the lowest GI, but you can use any low GI fruit you prefer.

**Time:** 5 minutes
**Serving Size:** 1
**Nutritional Facts:**
*Calories:* 240
*Carbs:* 13 g
*Sugar:* 10 g
*Fat:* 9 g
*Protein:* 24 g
**Ingredients:**
- 1 cup cottage cheese
- ½ cup cherries

**Directions:**

1. Wash the cherries and remove the stems. Cut cherries in half and discard the pits.

2. Add cottage cheese to a bowl and mix in cherry halves.

*Lunch - Grilled Basil Chicken*

Fresh herbs can really make a difference in recipes. This

recipe uses the natural flavor of basil to give the chicken a real punch.

**Time:** 10 minutes
**Serving Size:** 2
**Nutritional Facts:**
*Calories:* 412
*Carbs:* 1 g
*Sugar:* <1 g
*Fat:* 4 g
*Protein:* 37 g

**Ingredients:**
- ½ lb chicken breast, sliced thin
- 2 tbsp fresh basil, chopped
- 1 tbsp olive oil
- ¼ tsp salt
- ¼ tsp black pepper

**Directions:**

1. Add olive oil to a skillet and set the heat to medium-high. Lay out chicken breasts in a single layer and season with salt and pepper.

2. Cook chicken, flipping periodically until it is no longer pink in the center, about four minutes on each side.

3. Add basil and cook for another minute until flavor is well incorporated into the chicken.

*Snack - Garlic Roasted Edamame*

Edamame is a great source of protein. It makes for a quick and easy snack that can be easily enjoyed without much hassle.

**Time:** 15 minutes
**Serving Size:** 2
**Nutritional Facts:**
*Calories:* 198
*Carbs:* 7 g
*Sugar:* 3 g
*Fat:* 6 g

*Protein:* 12 g
**Ingredients:**
- 1 cup edamame
- 2 tbsp minced garlic
- 1 tbsp olive oil
- ½ tsp salt

**Directions:**

1. Bring water to boil in a pot over high heat. Add edamame and cook for five minutes until the beans are tender.

2. Heat olive oil in a skillet over medium heat. Add edamame and garlic and stir to coat. Cook until crispy, about 10 minutes, stirring frequently.

*Dinner - Leftovers*

You've made it through what is usually the most difficult period of the sugar detox. Give yourself a pat on the back by having leftovers for dinner. It's always a good idea to make extra servings with any recipe, knowing you'll have leftovers as a healthy and quick snack or meal option for later.

*Day Five*

Now that you've made use of fruit as a carb source, you can begin to include other sources. This primarily means whole grain bread products and brown rice. Adding in healthy carbs greatly expands the number of recipes available to you.

*Breakfast - Fried Eggs*

You can't go wrong with something simple like fried eggs. This recipe yields slightly runny yolks, but you can adjust the cooking time to your preference.

**Time:** 10 minutes
**Serving Size:** 1
**Nutritional Facts:**
*Calories:* 216
*Carbs:* 1 g
*Sugar:* <1 g
*Fat:* 15 g

*Protein:* 24 g
**Ingredients:**
- 3 eggs
- 1 tsp butter
- ½ tsp salt

**Directions:**

1. Heat butter in a pan over medium-high heat.

2. Crack eggs in the pan, keeping them separate from each other. When the bottom is firm, about three to four minutes, flip eggs. Cook for about three more minutes, then gently break the yolks and cook for a minute more until yolks are only semi-runny.

*Snack - Handful of Almonds*

No recipe needed for this snack. Simply take a serving of almonds in a bowl or reusable container and eat them on the go.

**Nutritional Facts:**
*Calories:* 115
*Carbs:* 4 g
*Sugar:* <1 g
*Fat:* 10 g
*Protein:* 6 g

*Lunch - Chickpea Salad*

Chickpeas prove their versatility once again by being a great addition to any salad. You can customize further by adding veggies of your choosing.

**Time:** 10 minutes
**Serving Size:** 1
**Nutritional Facts:**
*Calories:* 196
*Carbs:* 28 g
*Sugar:* 5 g
*Fat:* 3 g
*Protein:* 14 g
**Ingredients:**

- 8 oz chickpeas
- 2 cups romaine lettuce
- ½ bell pepper
- 1/4 cup shredded carrots

**Directions:**

1. Drain and rinse chickpeas. Chop up the lettuce and pepper.

2. Combine lettuce, chickpeas, pepper, and carrots in a bowl. Top with your choice of sugar-free dressing.

*Snack - Homemade Hummus*

Hummus pairs well with so many different veggies and whole grain snacks. Of course, it's also perfectly enjoyable on its own. You can make sure there's no added sugars in your hummus by making your own.

**Time:** 15 minutes

**Serving Size:** 6

**Nutritional Facts:**

*Calories:* 102

*Carbs:* 10 g

*Sugar:* 1 g

*Fat:* 3 g

*Protein:* 12 g

**Ingredients:**
- 15 oz chickpeas
- 1 lemon
- 1/4 cup tahini
- 2 tbsp minced garlic
- 2 tbsp olive oil
- ½ tsp ground cumin
- ½ tsp paprika

**Directions:**

1. Add tahini to a food processor. Cut and juice the lemon into the food processor, then blend for one minute, stirring halfway through.

2. Add garlic, olive oil, cumin, and paprika and pulse to mix. Slowly add in 1/4 cup of chickpeas at a time and process in 30 second intervals.

3. Thin hummus with water until desired consistency is reached.

*Dinner - Simple Garlic Chicken*

Sometimes less is more, and that's certainly the case with this garlic chicken!

**Time:** 15 minutes
**Serving Size:** 2
**Nutritional Facts:**
*Calories:* 396
*Carbs:* 1 g
*Sugar:* <1 g
*Fat:* 6 g
*Protein:* 56 g
**Ingredients:**
- ½ lb chicken breast, sliced thin
- 1 tsp butter
- 1 tsp garlic powder
- ½ tsp salt
- ½ tsp black pepper

**Directions:**
1. Melt butter in a skillet over medium heat.

2. Season chicken with garlic powder, salt, and black pepper. Add to the skillet and let cook for eight minutes, only disturbing to prevent sticking. Flip the chicken and cook for another eight minutes, letting the chicken get lightly crisped on both sides.

*Day Six*

Keep going strong with your commitment to the sugar detox. You are nearly at the end of the first week! Think about how far you have come and motivate yourself to keep going through all seven days.

*Breakfast - Strawberry and Coconut Yogurt Bowl*

Adding your own fruit to yogurt is the perfect way to get a source of natural sweetness to start off your morning. This yogurt bowl makes the most of this method for an amazing breakfast.

**Time:** 5 minutes
**Serving Size:** 1
**Nutritional Facts:**
*Calories:* 352
*Carbs:* 16 g
*Sugar:* 8 g
*Fat:* 11 g
*Protein:* 26 g

**Ingredients:**
- 1 cup Greek yogurt
- ¼ cup coconut milk
- 2 strawberries
- 1 tbsp shredded coconut
- 1 tbsp chia seeds

**Directions:**

1. In a medium bowl, add Greek yogurt and mix with coconut milk.

2. Wash and slice strawberries. Top yogurt with strawberry slices, shredded coconut, and chia seeds.

*Snack - Celery and Peanut Butter Sticks*

While the traditional "Ants-on-a-log" variant of this recipe uses raisins, we want to cut those out on our sugar detox. Instead, the celery and peanut butter alone still make for a delicious, healthy, and protein-filled snack.

**Time:** 5 minutes
**Serving Size:** 1
**Nutritional Fact/Info:**
*Calories:* 202
*Carbs:* 9 g

*Sugar:* 2 g
*Fat:* 15 g
*Protein:* 12 g
**Ingredients:**
- 4 celery sticks
- 2 tbsp unsweetened peanut butter

**Directions:**

*Lunch - Leftovers*

You've made nearly a week's worth of food, which means you probably have a fair number of leftovers already. Make good use of them to save yourself time during lunch.

*Snack - Berry Smoothie*

SMOOTHIES ARE JUST as good as snacks as they are for breakfast. Try this multi-berry smoothie for low GI fruits you can safely incorporate into your diet.

**Time:** 5 minutes
**Serving Size:** 1
**Nutritional Facts:**
*Calories:* 160
*Carbs:* 8 g
*Sugar:* 6 g
*Fat:* 2 g
*Protein:* 29 g
**Ingredients:**
- 1 cup coconut milk
- ½ cup strawberries, frozen
- ½ cup raspberries, frozen
- ¼ cup blueberries, frozen
- ⅓ cup protein powder
- ¼ cup spinach

**Directions:**

1. Add coconut milk, strawberries, raspberries, blueberries, protein powder, and spinach to a blender.

2. Pulse for 30-60 seconds until desired thickness is reached.

*Dinner - Tuscan Shrimp*

This shrimp recipe is sure to become a recurring staple of your dinner rotation. Pair it with riced cauliflower, brown rice, or just eat it as it is.

**Time:** 35 minutes
**Serving Size:** 2
**Nutritional Facts:**
*Calories:* 180
*Carbs:* 6 g
*Sugar:* 2 g
*Fat:* 5 g
*Protein:* 23 g

**Ingredients:**
- 2 lb shrimp, peeled and deveined
- 1 cup spinach, chopped
- ½ cup cherry tomatoes, diced
- ½ cup heavy cream
- ½ lemon
- 1 tbsp garlic, minced
- 1 tbsp olive oil

**Directions:**

1. Add olive oil to a skillet over medium-low heat. Lay shrimp in the pan and cook for about four minutes on each side, until shrimp are pink. Remove shrimp from the skillet and set aside.

2. Sauté garlic for one minute, then add cherry tomatoes and sauté for three minutes until soft. Mix in spinach and cook until spinach is wilted, then add shrimp and heavy cream.

3. Cook for another five minutes. Top with lemon juice and enjoy.

*Day Seven*

At this point, you can start to reintroduce zero-calorie sweeteners like Stevia into your diet. Keep the amount you use very low, but if you want to sweeten your coffee or have a small sugar-free dessert, that's okay too. Follow the last day of recipes to complete your first week on a sugar detox and finish strong.

*Breakfast - Avocado Toast with Cottage Cheese*

With whole grain bread, protein-packed avocados, and cottage cheese, this variant of avocado toast is especially tasty and energizing.

**Time:** 5 minutes
**Serving Size:** 1
**Nutritional Facts:**
*Calories:* 430
*Carbs:* 37 g
*Sugar:* 5 g
*Fat:* 16 g
*Protein:* 32 g

**Ingredients:**
- 2 slices whole grain bread
- ½ avocado
- ½ cup cottage cheese
- ½ tsp salt
- ¼ tsp pepper

**Directions:**
1. Toast bread to your desired preference.
2. While bread is toasting, slice the avocado open and remove the pit. Scoop out ½ of the avocado from its peel and slice.
3. Top the toast with cottage cheese and avocado. Sprinkle with salt and pepper and enjoy.

*Snack - Snap Peas and Hummus*

Snap peas are easy to eat while still getting work done. Adding hummus as a savory topping gives them a protein boost.

This recipe makes use of store-bought hummus, but you can always make your own using the recipe from day five.

**Time:** 5 minutes
**Serving Size:** 1
**Nutritional Facts:**
*Calories:* 262
*Carbs:* 24 g
*Sugar:* 2 g
*Fat:* 13 g
*Protein:* 14 g
**Ingredients:**
- 1 cup snap peas
- ½ cup plain hummus

**Directions:**

1. Clean snap peas by first rinsing and drying them. Slice the ends off of each pod, then remove the string that runs lengthwise down the pod.

2. Dip snap peas into hummus and enjoy.

*Lunch - Tuna Salad Sandwich*

Tuna has plenty of protein and great nutrients that are important for your diet. With whole grain bread, this sandwich is a great light lunch option.

**Time:** 15 minutes
**Serving Size:** 1
**Nutritional Facts:**
*Calories:* 444
*Carbs:* 28 g
*Sugar:* 4 g
*Fat:* 8 g
*Protein:* 49 g
**Ingredients:**
- 1 can of tuna
- 2 slices of whole grain bread
- 2 leaves of romaine lettuce

- 2 tbsp mayonnaise
- 1 stalk of celery, diced
- ½ lemon

**Directions:**

1. Drain tuna and transfer to a bowl. Mix with mayonnaise, celery, and the juice of half a lemon.

2. Layer tuna and lettuce on whole wheat bread, slice the sandwich in half, and enjoy.

*Snack - Wheat Crackers and Cheese*

If you need a quick snack, you can't go wrong with about five whole wheat crackers and some sliced cheddar cheese. These foods have minimal sugar and they are healthy sources of carbs.

**Nutritional Facts:**

*Calories:* 189

*Carbs:* 5 g

*Sugar:* 2 g

*Fat:* 9 g

*Protein:* 12 g

*Dinner - Leftovers*

Reward yourself for your diligent efforts by taking a break from cooking and enjoying something you made earlier in the week.

## REWARDS FOR COMPLETING WEEK ONE

You've just finished week one of your sugar detox diet! Even if you were dreading dropping sugar at the beginning of the week, you hopefully now see that you can still get the nutrition and energy you need without all of the negative health effects that sugar brings.

Since week one requires you to be so diligent in your restrictions, it is a good idea to reward yourself once you complete it. You don't want to go overboard, of course—this isn't an excuse to go back to cakes and cookies—but you can have some sugar-free treats made with zero-calorie sweeteners in moderation. Dessert should always be something you limit your consumption of, but it is okay to indulge when celebrating your first steps away from the control that sugar has held over your life for so long.

There are quite a few options for you to indulge in. After week one, it is okay to have up to three glasses of wine per week. You should space your glasses out so as not to introduce too much sugar into your system at once, and you should also avoid things like wine coolers and wine sweetened with other fruit beverages. These kinds of drinks are much higher in sugar than normal wine and will interfere with your goals, but the occasional glass is okay now that you have made it through the tough part.

If you've been craving chocolate, then dark chocolate and desserts made with unsweetened cocoa powder is acceptable. You should still avoid milk chocolate because it is packed with added sugars, but dark chocolate of at least 75% cacao is something sweet that won't ruin your progress. If you're used to milk chocolate, it can taste a little bitter at first, but this won't be a major issue for very long—the chocolate will win out in the end! Yogurt with a low GI fruit and a sprinkle of Stevia is a great option too.

MORE TRADITIONAL DESSERTS are still possible on a low-sugar diet so long as you are smart about your ingredients and make the desserts yourself rather than buying pre-made kinds. For example, there are many recipes for low-carb and high-protein cookies, cakes, cheesecakes, and brownies. These recipes typically use a zero-calorie sweetener, cocoa powder instead of milk chocolate, and low-carb alternatives to white flour such as almond flour and coconut flour. Even ice cream is possible if you blend some frozen, low-sugar fruits and yogurt together and chill the results. Be sure to check the ingredients of any recipe for hidden sources of sugar, but if you are vigilant about sugar, you can enjoy many of the desserts you did previously without any of the not-so-sweet consequences.

# 6

## STEP 5

### YOU WILL SLIP UP AND THAT'S OKAY

Despite our best intentions, sometimes we make mistakes and fail to live up to our own expectations. This can happen in any scenario, whether things don't quite go as planned at work or we fail to stick to our resolution to make healthier choices. When this happens, it is easy to pile guilt on yourself and turn to self-critical thoughts, but try to steer clear of this temptation. Guilt rarely works as an effective motivator, and more often than not just makes you believe the false idea that you cannot, or you are not strong enough to, change your eating habits. If you tell yourself that you will never change, and that your failure is a product of your "weakness," then you will have trouble recognizing just how strong you really can be. Give yourself the chance, and don't stop trying. The truth is that you are capable of succeeding no matter how many attempts it takes you. So long as you recognize that the sugar detox is hard, and offer yourself forgiveness when you falter, you will succeed.

A flawless sugar detox is very difficult, and maintaining a perfect detox is highly unlikely. You have probably been under sugar's thumb for years, if not decades of your life. To assume that your first attempt to escape it would be a complete success would be rather overconfident. Of course, this does not mean that you should give up and accept that you will be ruled by your desire for sugar forever. Instead, it means that you should accept small, temporary failures as part of the road towards success—to prevent them from becoming permanent failures. Learn to acknowledge your mistake, understand why you made the mistake, take steps to correct the behavior, and try again with your new knowledge and preparations. Your success on the sugar detox is not a matter of "if." It is a matter of "when." Taking a bit more time than you initially envisioned is nothing to be ashamed of. You are doing a difficult thing, but you are doing it for all the right reasons, and when you finally succeed you will feel more powerful for all of your initial struggles.

## HOW TO RECOVER FROM A MISSTEP

When you make a misstep on your sugar detox by giving in to your cravings and eating high in sugar, you don't want to punish yourself for the mistake, but you don't want it to continue uncorrected either. Here are some steps you can employ to minimize the risk of future mistakes while still keeping yourself motivated to keep trying to separate yourself from sugar.

*Recognize Your Mistake*

You can't fix a mistake if you don't acknowledge that it happened. It's tempting to brush off small slip-ups. You may say to yourself, "Yes, I had a piece of candy, but so what? It was only a few grams of sugar and I doubt that it made much of a difference," or, "I didn't realize what I was eating was high in sugar until it was too late. But it wasn't my fault." However, trying to rationalize and excuse the behavior only makes it more likely to reoccur. If you give yourself a free pass this time, what's to say you won't give yourself another one next time? You can hardly hold yourself accountable for your eating choices if you brush every mistake under the rug. First and foremost, accept and own the fact that you ate or drank something you weren't supposed to.

*Let the Guilt Go*

Once you acknowledge your mistake, feelings of guilt may start to creep up. You may punish yourself for what you did, even if the mistake was relatively minor or unintentional. This is especially common if negative emotions were what drove you towards sugar. The last thing you want to do is make yourself so guilty that the only way you can deal with that feeling is to eat sugar again. If you allow guilty feelings to fester, they will discourage you from giving the sugar detox another shot. You'll think, "I already messed up once, so I'll probably do it again, which means there's no point in trying to stop eating sugar." This is a defeatist attitude that only ensures you really will never be able to make a change. If you avoid feeling guilty and instead think positively about your future attempts, you will give yourself the motivation you need to try again, this time with more commitment to not caving to cravings.

*Identify the Trigger*

There was a reason why, despite good intentions, you returned to sugar. What was it? This will be different for everyone and is often affected by the day's circumstances. For example, maybe you had an especially difficult day, or maybe you got a poor night of sleep. Perhaps you had a very specific craving because of a certain location or activity that reminded you of previous times eating a certain sugary food. Figuring out what triggered your intense, irresistible desire for sugar requires a bit of introspection, but only through considering your behaviors and thought process can you ensure the mistake doesn't happen again.

*Avoid Making the Same Mistake Again*

Now that you know what event or circumstance causes you to reach for sugar, you can ensure you avoid it going forward.

The steps you take to avoid the trigger will depend on what your particular trigger is. If a lack of sleep made you more tired than usual, try to make sure you are going to bed and waking up in regular patterns. This kind of change makes it less likely that you will encounter that trigger again. If you had a bad day or encountered something upsetting, see if there are any behaviors other than sugar that you can use to release tension and improve your mood. Maybe this means working out your frustration, or maybe it means watching a TV show you enjoy or hanging out with friends to soothe your emotions. Next time when you encounter the trigger that caused you to eat sugar, you will be able to work around it.

## CHOOSE SMALL SUGAR ALLOWANCES OVER FULL BINGES

When you slip up, you may be tempted to just throw in the towel. Since you've already made one mistake for the day, why not get your fill of sugar and just restart everything tomorrow? This mentality can manifest when cravings get really bad. A fair option here is to allow yourself a single piece of candy or something similar. This soothes your craving but leaves you space to think about the repercussions of your action. The danger is that if you resist even the smallest allowance of sugar for so long, when you do finally cave, you may go all-out and binge on sugar.

It is better to have one small slip-up that is quickly course corrected than to stuff yourself with sugar. You will find it easier to get back to your sugar detox if you allow yourself something small in an effort to avoid a much bigger binge. You don't want to cave to every slight craving, of course, but you also don't want cravings to get so bad that you completely derail your progress when they overpower you.

The sugar detox is not just a single week of changes before

you go back to your regular eating habits. There is no end point, after which you will be able to keep eating sugar without repercussions. The goal is an entirely new habit that will lead to a healthier life overall. You will need to make some difficult decisions and negotiate your cravings, and that means sometimes doing damage control to avoid sugar binges. You are most likely going to be dealing with tough cravings for a long time, perhaps months and even years into the future. Learn when to hold firm in the face of sugar's temptations and when it is better to make a sort of compromise with your cravings—satisfy them with a small bit of sugar if they promise to let you go back to not craving sugar right after. Building these systems for craving management in the long-term ensures that you never return to the excessive overconsumption of sugar.

## FOCUS ON YOUR MOTIVATION

Motivation can mean the difference between success and failure. It is what keeps you going in the most difficult times and what convinces you to try again if you make a mistake. Without a source of motivation, your desire to make any change in your life is minimal. You might start a sugar detox, but your willpower to see it through and to maintain the change will waver very quickly, and you will find yourself right back where you started.

Not every source of motivation is the same. Some will successfully encourage you with positive thoughts of the life you could have if you cut your ties to sugar, while others motivate you through fear of what sugar will do to your body or what others will think of you. It is okay to have a little of each of these types of motivations influencing your decision to quit sugar. After all, the health conditions accelerated by sugar are legitimately dangerous. But in general, positive and internal motivators are far more effective than negative and external ones. Consider what you really want to achieve and, more importantly than that, why you want to achieve it. The reason why you are trying to make a change can be the most powerful motivator of all.

*Weight Loss Vs. Long-Term Health*

People start diets for all sorts of reasons. Perhaps the most common is the desire to lose weight. This isn't always a bad thing, as excess weight has a negative impact on your health, but it is often a somewhat weaker motivation because it is tied to an external factor rather than an internal one. Think about why you want to lose weight. Is it to make yourself healthy, or is it to improve others' opinions of you? Are you trying to lose weight because you don't want to face ridicule, or perhaps because others have told you that you need to in the past, whether they are doctors or not? These motivators come from the desire to avoid negative outcomes. If you find dissatisfaction in your appearance and want to lose weight because of it, you are likely to remain dissatisfied and self-critical whether you lose weight or not. This can make it hard to stick to a diet, because the outcome that matters most—how you feel about yourself—will not change no matter how little sugar you eat.

If you want a truly powerful motivator, look for one that comes from trying to achieve a positive outcome rather than avoid a negative one. The difference may seem minimal, but when you shoot for a positive outcome, you are working hard because you, personally, want something. You are more driven and focused because the outcome matters more to you. You are working for your own goals, not because of others' opinions or a critical view of yourself. You are actively trying to improve yourself in a way that makes you feel good because you know you are setting yourself up for a longer, happier life. This will give you the motivation you need to commit yourself to the sugar detox.

## FORGIVE YOURSELF AND SET YOURSELF UP FOR FUTURE SUCCESS

After you've identified your mistake, you must show yourself forgiveness. You can spend days or weeks getting frustrated with yourself or feeling guilty, or you can move forward with your sugar detox and try again, but you cannot do the latter effectively without forgiving yourself for what went wrong. Detoxing from sugar is going to be hard, and there will be moments where you want to quit entirely. Guilt and criticism only make it more likely that you will decide the effort is not worth the results. You give yourself an incredible advantage by accepting that some mistakes will occur, but you do not have to let them keep you down for long.

After forgiving yourself, move forward with a plan to do better the next day. You can make this process easier on yourself by following a pre-made meal plan, which takes a lot of the guesswork and stress out of trying to find foods that meet your needs each day. Use the meal plan to help you prep your meals in advance if time is something that keeps you from succeeding. If you tend to grab something quick and not so nutritious when you get home from a long day of work, prep your meals on your days off instead so you only have to heat them up throughout the week. Additionally, make sure you are getting adequate nutrition from your weekly meals. If you are left with big calorie deficits every day, chances are your cravings will be much worse as well. Drinking plenty of water helps you stay hydrated and feel full as well, and staying busy can reduce the time you have to daydream about cakes and cookies.

*Support and Accountability*

Sometimes all you need is a little support from those around you. Feeling like others are invested in your success encourages you to give the sugar detox your full effort. Sharing your plan with family members and friends means you are making an effort to change your habits and they can support that effort—you're not going this alone. There are now others who are expecting you to follow the plan you have laid out and they can hold you accountable for this in a supportive way. It also means they are more likely to accommodate your new diet if you get together for lunch, so there will be sugar-free options available and you will be less likely to cheat the detox.

Having someone else to do the sugar detox with is another amazing way to keep yourself motivated. Check in and see if any of your friends and family members are interested in cutting sugar out of their diets. It is much easier to stick to a new diet if everyone in your household is eating under the same guidelines. You can completely remove unhealthy foods from the house rather than having to keep them around for other family members, and you can share healthy meals that the whole family will enjoy. Having to watch those around you eat restricted foods is tough, and it increases the chances of you deciding you will have "just one bite" of the offending food. Stay strong, approach healthy eating as a group effort, and you will be much more likely to stick to your sugar detox.

## 7

## THE DETOX IS DONE. NOW WHAT?

You have now completed your sugar detox. It was likely difficult to retrain your brain, and you probably had a few stumbling blocks and delays, but you stuck to it and effectively eliminated excess sugars from your diet. What's next? Do you go back to how you ate before, or do you carry on practicing the habits you learned and continue eating with your newfound freedom from sugar in mind?

First, take a moment to think of all the positive results you have made for yourself. After my own sugar detox, I eased my reliance on sugar to cope with emotional struggles. I found healthier ways to deal with the trauma I endured at a young age. I learned skills that helped me start healing from that painful time rather than simply soothing my symptoms with sugar. I was able to focus and address the root of my problem. As a result of this, I lost a great deal of weight by ditching the unhealthy coping habits I had developed over years of practice. I avoided many of the difficult, painful, and scary health conditions that come with excessive weight and excessive sugar consumption. I effectively turned my life around. You have likely noticed the beginnings of similar changes in yourself. In order to receive the full benefits of a life free from sugar addiction, you must continue practicing the healthy eating habits you have learned and never fall back into sugar's trap again.

## YOUR NEXT STEPS

The sugar detox includes a more active phase, where you take steps to consciously reduce your sugar and slowly start to reintroduce carbs. After you have completed this step, you only need to continue practicing what you have learned. You cannot go right back to eating sugar, nor is it a good idea to eat foods you know to be unhealthy, even if they aren't strictly prohibited with the looser restrictions you are now following. Continue to make smart, healthy choices and give yourself the greatest advantages you can.

*Keep Carb Sources Healthy*

It's okay to eat carbs, but make sure you're getting them from whole foods and other natural sources. Not all carbs are good for you. You can eat whole wheat pasta and whole grain bread, but finishing your sugar detox is no excuse to rush to McDonald's to get a burger, fries, and soda.

Sugars that naturally occur in whole grains, vegetables, and some fruits are okay, while less healthy alternatives should be avoided. Remember to check the glycemic index (GI) of any sugary fruit before eating it, and if you do eat something high in sugar, try to limit your consumption. For example, stick to one half rather than having a whole apple. Carbs in general are perfectly fine, but carbs that negatively impact your blood sugar and cause it to spike can send you back into a sugar addiction over time.

*Continue to Restrict Added Sugars*

Naturally occurring sugars are okay to reintroduce into

your diet, even from sources like sweet fruits, but you should still limit or entirely restrict the amount of added sugar you eat. Added sugars directly interfere with any food's health benefits and greatly increase the chance of falling back into sugar addiction. You can avoid them by limiting your consumption of prepackaged food and pre-made meals, instead choosing whole ingredients without sauces and added flavorings.

The one exception to this is zero-calorie sweeteners, which can generally be used without too much risk of triggering your sugar addiction once again. They do not affect your blood sugar levels, so they don't cause your energy or mood to spike quite as dangerously as other sources of sugar. They are okay to consume in moderate amounts, though you should still prioritize whole foods.

*Stick to Homemade Meals as Often as Possible*

The sugar detox likely made you more familiar with cooking your own meals if you tended to buy pre-made meals previously. This is a good habit to maintain after the detox. When making your own meals, you get to decide exactly what goes into them and what doesn't make the cut. You can leave added sugars out of the picture and only buy ingredients that are well suited for a low sugar lifestyle. The meals you make will be completely free of harmful additives so you can be sure you are serving yourself and your family a healthy meal that you can be proud of.

For busy weeks, make use of meal prep on the weekends, or use a slow cooker to have a meal ready to eat by the time you get home. There are also many quick, simple meals you can make without much time commitment. A sliced protein cooks much faster than a whole chicken breast or steak, and pan-frying is typically quicker than baking. If you throw together a sliced protein, some diced vegetables, and brown rice that you cooked in bulk on the weekends, you can have a healthy and filling stir-fry in as little as 20 minutes. Egg dishes also cook very quickly, as do most seafood options. Cooking for yourself on a tight schedule is not nearly as difficult as it sounds at first.

## MONITOR YOUR SWEET TOOTH

It's important to recognize that sugar may continue to be a temptation even after the sugar detox is done. You may not be addicted to sugar any longer, but if you indulge in it too often, you can build up the same habits that led to addiction in the first place and need to go through the detox all over again. Still, over time your cravings for sugar will lessen as you put distance between sugar and yourself. The longer you resist going back to sugar, the easier it will be to continue doing so.

That being said, it is okay to have a little bit of sugar here and there so long as sugar does not control your eating habits. Many people are able to have a healthy relationship with sugar, even after being trapped in a sugar addiction. It's alright to have a few bites of cake at a birthday party or to reward yourself with a sugary drink every once in a while, but try to keep the overall level of sugar you consume to a minimum. Continue checking labels and keeping an eye out for hidden sugars so you don't slip back into old habits without even realizing your sugar consumption is increasing.

You can help limit the amount of sugar you consume by looking for new, exciting recipes every day. There are thousands of low-carb and low-sugar recipes. Trying something new keeps your excitement for food high, even when these foods have next to no sugar in them. The culinary world is immense, filled with uncountable recipes that taste amazing without putting your health in jeopardy. Make use of all recipes available to you and keep your meals varied so you never have to resort to sugar for a quick mood boost ever again.

# AFTERWORD

Learning to separate yourself from sugar isn't always an easy choice to make. It is usually one that requires you to confront the reality of just how heavily sugar has impacted your life and your health. If you use sugar as a crutch for dealing with emotional distress, part of the detox process involves looking at the behaviors and situations that trigger sugar cravings and finding ways to deal with these issues. Despite its difficulty, leaving your sugar addiction behind is always worth the effort, and you will experience a much higher quality of life when you are no longer dependent on sugar for happiness.

Throughout this book, you have learned all of the ways sugar can sneak into your diet—and the steps you must take to ensure added sugars are banned from your kitchen. You have seen the importance of alternatives like complex carbohydrates and protein. You have given yourself the tools for sugar detox success on a sugar detox, including a meal plan, positive motivators for your new diet, and the strength to deal with slip-ups. All that is left is for you to put this information into practice.

You are fully capable of cutting sugar and all of its negative health repercussions. It will take some trial and error, and there

## AFTERWORD

may be moments when you are tempted to give up on your attempt, but if you keep motivated and try again you will get to enjoy all of the health benefits of a sugar-free lifestyle. Live a healthier, happier life, and move on from your sugar addiction.

If you found this book to be beneficial in your journey to lessen your reliance on sugar, consider giving it a positive review. This helps others benefit from the sugar detox, letting many people learn how to take back control of their diets—just as you have.

# REFERENCES

AlexanderStein. (2013, Sept. 19). *Dark chocolate.* Pixabay. https://pixabay.com/photos/chocolate-dark-coffee-confiserie-183543/

Arnarson, A. (2017, Feb. 1). *8 surprising health benefits of edamame.* Healthline. https://www.healthline.com/nutrition/edamame-benefits#section3

ArtCoreStudios. (2016, Dec. 29). *Banana pancakes.* Pixabay. https://pixabay.com/photos/pancakes-banana-breakfast-food-1931089/

Congerdesign. (2014, Dec. 20). *Mixed vegetables.* Pixabay. https://pixabay.com/photos/vegetables-knife-paprika-573961/

Cox, L. (2013, May 30). *Why is too much salt bad for you?* Live Science. https://www.livescience.com/36256-salt-bad-health.html

Difisher. (2018, June 16). *Kitchen pantry.* Pixabay. https://pixabay.com/photos/fridge-fridge-door-refrigerator-3475996/

Djanoff. (2018, July 5). *Roasted chickpeas.* Pixabay. https://pixabay.com/photos/roasted-chickpeas-healthy-recipes-3516806/

Harrar, S. (2019, Mar. 29). *Insulin resistance causes and symp-*

*toms*. EndocrineWeb. https://www.endocrineweb.com/conditions/type-2-diabetes/insulin-resistance-causes-symptoms

Harvard Health Publishing. (2020, Jan. 6). *Glycemic index for 60+ foods*. https://www.health.harvard.edu/diseases-and-conditions/glycemic-index-and-glycemic-load-for-100-foods

Johnson, J. (2018, Sept. 26). *What to know about diet soda and diabetes*. Medical News Today. https://www.medicalnewstoday.com/articles/310909#diet-soda-and-diabetes

Murray, K. (2020, Apr. 29). *Sugar addiction*. Addiction Center. https://www.addictioncenter.com/drugs/sugar-addiction/

Oldmermaid. (2016, Feb. 8). *White flour pasta*. Pixabay. https://pixabay.com/photos/pasta-fettuccine-food-italian-1181189/

Pexels. (2017, Mar. 27). *Healthy carbs*. Pixabay. https://pixabay.com/photos/bread-breakfast-dinner-wholesome-2178874/

PhotoMIX-Company. (2016, May 24). *Strawberry smoothie*. Pixabay. https://pixabay.com/photos/strawberry-drink-kefir-the-drink-1411374/

Puscas, C. (2018, Feb. 13). *9 high-protein foods that will kill your sugar cravings*. Feedr. https://blog.feedr.co/blog/9-high-protein-foods-to-kill-sugar-cravings/

Santos-Longhurst, A. (2018, Nov. 26). *How to beat sugar detox symptoms and feel better than ever*. Healthline. https://www.healthline.com/health/sugar-detox-symptoms

Stevepb. (2016, Aug. 25). *Dairy products*. Pixabay. https://pixabay.com/photos/refrigerator-fridge-cold-storage-1619676/

Wow_Pho. (2016, Apr. 21). *Grilled chicken and salad*. Pixabay. https://pixabay.com/photos/grilled-chicken-quinoa-salad-1334632/

www.ingramcontent.com/pod-product-compliance
Lightning Source LLC
Chambersburg PA
CBHW031157020426
42333CB00013B/716